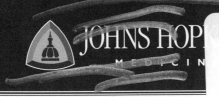

Patients' Guide to
Head and Neck Cancer

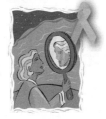

Christine G. Gourin, MD, FACS
Associate Professor
Director, Clinical Research Program in Head and Neck Cancer
Department of Otolaryngology-Head and Neck Surgery
Johns Hopkins University
Baltimore, MD

SERIES EDITORS
Lillie D. Shockney, RN, BS, MAS
University Distinguished Service Associate Professor of Breast Cancer; Administrative Director of Breast Cancer; Associate Professor, Department of Surgery; Associate Professor, Department of Obstetrics and Gynecology, Johns Hopkins School of Medicine; Associate Professor, Johns Hopkins School of Nursing

Gary R. Shapiro, MD
Chairman, Department of Oncology
Johns Hopkins Bayview Medical Center
Director, Johns Hopkins Geriatric Oncology Program
The Sidney Kimmel Comprehensive Cancer Center at Johns Hopkins

JONES & BARTLETT
L E A R N I N G

World Headquarters
Jones & Bartlett Learning
40 Tall Pine Drive
Sudbury, MA 01776
978-443-5000
info@jblearning.com
www.jblearning.com

Jones & Bartlett Learning
Canada
6339 Ormindale Way
Mississauga, Ontario L5V 1J2
Canada

Jones & Bartlett Learning
International
Barb House, Barb Mews
London W6 7PA
United Kingdom

Jones & Bartlett Learning books and products are available through most bookstores and online booksellers. To contact Jones & Bartlett Learning directly, call 800-832-0034, fax 978-443-8000, or visit our website, www.jblearning.com.

Substantial discounts on bulk quantities of Jones & Bartlett Learning publications are available to corporations, professional associations, and other qualified organizations. For details and specific discount information, contact the special sales department at Jones & Bartlett Learning via the above contact information or send an email to specialsales@jblearning.com.

The authors, editor, and publisher have made every effort to provide accurate information. However, they are not responsible for errors, omissions, or for any outcomes related to the use of the contents of this book and take no responsibility for the use of the products and procedures described. Treatments and side effects described in this book may not be applicable to all people; likewise, some people may require a dose or experience a side effect that is not described herein. Drugs and medical devices are discussed that may have limited availability controlled by the Food and Drug Administration (FDA) for use only in a research study or clinical trial. Research, clinical practice, and government regulations often change the accepted standard in this field. When consideration is being given to use of any drug in the clinical setting, the healthcare provider or reader is responsible for determining FDA status of the drug, reading the package insert, and reviewing prescribing information for the most up-to-date recommendations on dose, precautions, and contraindications, and determining the appropriate usage for the product. This is especially important in the case of drugs that are new or seldom used.

Production Credits
Executive Publisher: Christopher Davis
Editorial Assistant: Sara Cameron
Production Editor: Daniel Stone
Senior Marketing Manager: Alisha Weisman
V.P., Manufacturing and Inventory Control: Therese Connell
Cover Design: Kristin E. Parker
Cover Image: © ImageZoo/age fotostock
Composition: Auburn Associates, Inc.
Printing and Binding: Malloy, Inc.
Cover Printing: Malloy, Inc.

Library of Congress Cataloging-in-Publication Data
Gourin, Christine G.
  The Johns Hopkins patients' guide to head and neck cancer / Christine Gourin.
    p. cm.
  Includes bibliographical references and index.
  ISBN-13: 978-0-7637-7431-8
  ISBN-10: 0-7637-7431-6
  1. Head—Cancer—Popular works. 2. Neck—Cancer—Popular works. I. Title. II. Title: Patients' guide to head and neck cancer.
  RC280.H4G68 2010
  616.99'491—dc22

                                        2009019591

6048

Printed in the United States of America
14 13 12 11 10   10 9 8 7 6 5 4 3 2 1

TABLE OF CONTENTS

Contributors

Erin J. Blume, BS, RHIA
Clinic Manager, Department of Radiation Oncology &
    Molecular Radiation Sciences
The Sidney Kimmel Comprehensive Cancer Center at
    Johns Hopkins
Baltimore, MD

Christine G. Gourin, MD, FACS
Associate Professor
Director, Clinical Research Program in Head and
    Neck Cancer
Department of Otolaryngology–Head and Neck Surgery
Johns Hopkins University
Baltimore, MD

Carol S. Maragos, MSN, CRNP, CNOR
Nurse Practioner, Department of Otolaryngology–
    Head and Neck Surgery
Johns Hopkins University
Baltimore, MD

Gary R. Shapiro, MD
Chairman, Department of Oncology
Johns Hopkins Bayview Medical Center
Director, Johns Hopkins Geriatric Oncology Program
The Sidney Kimmel Comprehensive Cancer Center at
    Johns Hopkins
Baltimore, MD

Heather M. Starmer, MA, MS, CCC-SLP
Assistant Professor, Department of Otolaryngology–
    Head and Neck Surgery
Johns Hopkins University
Baltimore, MD

Kimberly Webster, MA, MS, CCC-SLP
Assistant Professor, Department of Otolaryngology–
    Head and Neck Surgery
Johns Hopkins University
Adjunct Faculty Member
University of Maryland and Towson University
Baltimore, MD

PREFACE

Over 40,000 new cases of head and neck cancer are diagnosed annually in the United States, which makes the patient with head and neck cancer a member of a large and growing community. Empowering yourself is the key to making informed decisions, participating in treatment choices presented to you by your oncology team, and gaining confidence that you are on the right track as you embark on this journey.

This is a time of increasing hope and excitement in the head and neck cancer community. New therapies have emerged in the past few years, leading to progressive improvements in both survival and quality of life for people with this type of cancer. Advances include studies showing that chemotherapy may improve survival when included as part of the treatment in people with high risk tumors, and the development of novel targeted therapies that may improve survival in patients with advanced disease. There have been major improvements in radiation and surgical approaches that lead to fewer side effects and better outcomes.

One of the most important aspects of head and neck cancer treatment in the 21st century is the team, or multidisciplinary approach, to care. The newly diagnosed patient quickly becomes the central member of a large team, including professionals from various disciplines who work together to determine the right therapy options for a particular patient. The authorship of this book reflects the diversity of this team, drawing from many disciplines that comprise the head and neck cancer program at Johns Hopkins.

This book is part of a series of Johns Hopkins Cancer Patient Guides designed to educate newly diagnosed patients about their cancer diagnosis and the treatment that may lie ahead. This book is not meant to be an exhaustive resource but rather an introduction to a diagnosis of head and neck cancer, written for patients and their families and friends. Reading may prompt more questions than answers. All questions are good questions; write them down and use this book as a starting point for conversations with your healthcare providers about your options.

It is my hope that you find this information useful. I wish you much success on this journey.

Christine G. Gourin, MD, FACS

Introduction

How to Use This Book to Your Benefit

Yͦou will receive a great deal of information from your healthcare team. You will also probably seek out some information on the Internet or in bookstores. No doubt friends and family members, meaning well, will offer you advice on what to do and when to do it, and will try to steer you in certain directions. Relax. Yes, you have heard words you wish you had never heard said about you, that you have head and neck cancer. Despite that shocking phrase, you have time to make good decisions and to empower yourself with accurate information so that you can participate in the decision making about your care and treatment.

This book is designed to be a how-to guide that will take you through the maze of treatment options and sometimes complicated schedules, and will help you put together a plan of action so that you become a head and neck cancer survivor.

The majority of patients diagnosed today will be survivors of this disease. Your goal is to join that majority.

This book is broken down into chapters and includes an index as well as credible resources listed for your further review and education. By empowering yourself with understandable information, we hope you will be comfortable participating in the decision making about your treatment.

You don't need to rush into treatment immediately. You have time on your side to plan things well and confidently.

Let's begin now with understanding what has happened and what the steps are to get you well again.

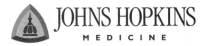

FIRST STEPS—I'VE BEEN DIAGNOSED WITH HEAD AND NECK CANCER

Christine G. Gourin, MD, FACS

Y ou may have recently had a biopsy of a neck mass that showed cancer or been told by a physician that the pain in your throat or change in your voice is due to a growth that looks like cancer. No doubt you are in shock after hearing those words. It is common for people to think, "How did this happen to me?" and even more common to think of a diagnosis of head and neck cancer as a death sentence. Because these are uncommon tumors, accounting for only 4% of all cancers, there is not much information available compared to more common cancers such as breast and colon cancer. Let's begin with answering some common questions.

RISK FACTORS

Risk factors for head and neck cancer include a history of tobacco use or alcohol abuse, or both in combination. These risk factors are present in 75% of patients diagnosed with head and neck cancer, with the exception of thyroid cancer. Other risk factors include a history of radiation to the head and neck. In the 1950s, this type of radiation was commonly used to treat acne or enlarged adenoids, and currently is used as part of the treatment of cancers of the head and neck. We are learning that some people who do not have any of these risk factors do have a history of human papillomavirus (HPV) infection, and we think that HPV may actually cause many cases of cancer of the tonsil and base of the tongue. Thyroid cancer occurs in 1 in 10 people with thyroid nodules or a goiter. This association is even stronger in men, those with rapidly growing nodules, or previous radiation exposure. Finally, a history of head and neck cancer in a family member is associated with a fourfold increase in risk of developing a head and neck cancer.

Only about 15% to 20% of patients diagnosed with head and neck cancer have a family history—meaning most patients have no family history at all. Sometimes people assume that a family history of cancer of any kind is the same thing as a history of head and neck cancer in the family, but this is not true. According to the American Cancer Society, one in three people in the United States will develop some type of cancer in their lifetime. There are certain cancers that carry a potential genetic link. Breast, ovarian, melanoma, pancreatic, and thyroid cancers can run in families and should trigger a discussion with a genetics counselor.

By and large, most patients who are diagnosed with head and neck cancer have no familial history that predisposed them to getting this disease.

There are some risk factors patients have that we simply don't know exist yet, and this is the focus of ongoing research. Trying to guess them will exhaust you and use up energy that is better saved for your fight against cancer.

LEARNING ABOUT YOUR DISEASE BEFORE THE FIRST VISIT

The first step in learning about your disease is determining what kind of cancer you have as well as what area of the head and neck is involved. Keep in mind that the earlier you are diagnosed, the better the chance for cure and the less treatment you will need to become a long-term survivor. Early-stage cancer (cancer which has not spread to lymph nodes and is small) can be treated successfully with single modality therapy in the form of surgery or radiation, depending on the tumor cell type and the site involved. Advanced stage cancer usually requires what is called multimodality therapy (more than one kind of treatment). This can consist of surgery followed by radiation therapy, or radiation therapy combined with chemotherapy. These are only rough guidelines, as different tumor types and characteristics may lead your doctor to add chemotherapy to surgery and radiation, or in the case of lymphoma, chemotherapy alone. Newer surgical techniques can preserve as much normal tissue as possible to minimize the impact of surgery on speech, swallowing, or shoulder function. Today, many patients are candidates for conservation surgery, which spares as much normal tissue as possible and may permit lower doses of radiation to be used post-operatively or avoid the use of radiation altogether.

Searching the Internet will yield a bewildering array of information, not all of which is accurate and some of which may be upsetting. Before you search for information from the Internet, journals, or books, the most important first step is for you to seek medical advice from a qualified head and neck oncologist. There is always more than one option for untreated patients, and you need to learn about all of the treatment options for your tumor type and stage before searching for information from other sources such as the Internet, journals, and books. This will save you the effort of poring through information which may not pertain to your particular situation.

Research shows that patients who seek emotional support during and after treatment have higher survival rates than those who decline to do so. The side effects from adjuvant treatment (chemotherapy and radiation) can be minimized with the use of drugs now available for that purpose. The side effects of surgery and radiation can be overcome by working with a speech pathologist and physical therapist during and after treatment. The majority of people are able to work and continue their activities of daily living during treatment.

GATHERING RECORDS: BIOPSY, RADIOLOGY STUDIES, AND OTHER TESTS

As soon as you hear the word "cancer," you should request a copy of the pathologist's biopsy report as well as any X-rays or imaging studies you have had done recently. This could be an ultrasound, CT scan, MRI, or PET scan. No matter who sees you—surgeon, medical oncologist or radiation oncologist—they will want to review these tests. They also need to see the actual films or images taken, not just the report. Ask the facility where the imaging was done how you can obtain the actual films. You should pick these up and hand carry them with you to your first consultation visit. The same is true for the actual pathology slides from your biopsy. You might wonder why you need to get these if they have the reports. The answer is that an accredited cancer center is required to review the images and the pathology slides to verify their accuracy. There are situations in which an error is discovered on a review by a head and neck pathologist who specializes in this disease. Sometimes the pathologist finds that the patient doesn't have cancer but instead has a condition that can mimic cancer. Another scenario is that the initial review suggested invasive cancer when a head and neck pathologist finds that it is noninvasive disease (or vice versa). Either way, these results could change the treatment dramatically. At every step your treatment plan is based on this information being correct. Be sure to obtain copies of all of your medical records and request copies as you continue this journey so you can maintain your own portfolio of your care and treatment and test results.

HOW TO SELECT YOUR ONCOLOGY TEAM

Your first chance to treat cancer is your best chance to cure it. Make sure you are putting yourself in the hands of experts. This isn't a simple gallbladder problem or hernia repair. Don't rely on self-promoting advertisements on television as a way to select a facility and doctor. Seek out a comprehensive cancer center that is NCI-designated (National Cancer Institute). To find an NCI-designated cancer center, go to www.cancer.gov. Such a facility will have fellowship-trained head and neck surgical oncologists (who are different from general surgeons who do some head and neck surgeries as well as some hernia operations and appenctomies), head and neck medical oncologists, head and neck radiation oncologists, head and neck pathologists, head and neck imaging radiologists, genetics counselors, oncology nurses, speech pathologists who specialize in voice and swallowing rehabilitation, and psychosocial support staff for head and neck cancer patients. This is a highly specialized group that works together to provide comprehensive cancer care.

Studies have confirmed that having your treatment done by cancer specialists gives you a higher probability of survival than having it done by generalists. For example, if you are seeing a surgeon to whom your family doctor referred you, ask questions.

- How many head and neck cancer surgeries does he or she do a year?

- What percentage of their patients get non-operative therapy and what percentage undergo surgery? (Not every cancer or patient is appropriate for non-operative therapy).

- What other types of surgeries does he or she perform and, therefore, how much of their time is spent doing head and neck cancer treatment? (You don't want a "cancer dabbler" or a "jack of all trades and master of none").

- Is he or she board certified? In what field?

- How long has he or she been in practice?

- Does he or she regularly attend head and neck cancer tumor boards to present cases for team discussion?

- Does he or she work with a multidisciplinary team of oncologists, nurses, and speech pathologists who specialize in head and neck cancer, so continuity of care and communication about your progress can be maintained?

- What is his or her philosophy on educating patients about their treatment options?

- How many sentinel node biopsies has he or she performed?

- Does he or she have photographs of patients they have operated on so you can see what the incisions look like and what reconstructive options there are?

These are all questions that you have the right to have answers to before deciding on a head and neck surgical oncologist. If he or she hesitates when answering any of your questions, this may be a sign that you do not want this particular doctor to be in charge of your care and helping you fight your fight against head and neck cancer.

It is not unusual for patients to get a second opinion after an initial consultation, particularly if they have initially gone to a small facility where head and neck oncology specialists may not be available. Your doctor should encourage and assist you in seeking a second opinion if you ask about this. Hesitation or refusal should also be a warning sign to you that this doctor may not be the best individual to direct your cancer treatment.

Head and Neck Cancer Sites

Head and neck cancer can arise from a variety of organs and sites, some of which you may not have heard of before. These include:

*   *Skin* (all skin involving the head and neck area, including the face, scalp, ears, and neck).

*   *Nasal cavity* (nose).

*   *Sinuses* (air-filled spaces behind your cheeks, nose, and forehead).

*   *Nasopharynx* (the area behind the nose at the base of the skull, above the roof of your mouth).

*   *Oral cavity* (the gums, lips, tongue, area under the tongue or floor of mouth, palate, or roof of the mouth).

*   *Oropharynx* (tonsils, base of the tongue, back wall of the throat at the level of the tongue, the soft palate and uvula).

*   *Larynx* ("voice box"—the true vocal cords, false vocal cords above the true vocal cords, epiglottis or valve above the vocal cords that protects you from food being swallowed into your lungs, and the trachea or windpipe immediately below the vocal cords, with surrounding cartilage ["Adam's apple"]).

*   *Hypopharynx* (the back wall of the digestive tract below the tongue and behind the larynx, including

the upper part of the esophagus, also called the cervical esophagus).

- *Trachea* (starts below the larynx; is a passage for air to the lungs).

- *Esophagus* (starts just below the larynx and carries food through the chest to the stomach. The cervical esophagus, which is the upper-third of the esophagus, is considered part of the head and neck).

- *Salivary glands* (the parotid glands, submandibular glands, and minor salivary glands lining the mouth and throat).

- *Thyroid gland* (a butterfly-shaped gland in the lower neck, in front of the larynx, which makes thyroid hormone, important in metabolism).

- *Lymph nodes* (there are hundreds of lymph nodes in both sides of the neck; these contain lymphatic tissue, which filter foreign substances and make white blood cells). Cancer may spread to lymph nodes, which is a sign of more advanced disease.

- *Neck* (in addition to lymph nodes, the neck contains blood vessels and nerves which may give rise to a variety of unusual tumor types).

CANCER STAGING

Staging is the most important part of your workup following a diagnosis of cancer. Initially, all information printed on medical reports and told to you will sound like Greek. By the end of your treatment you will be quoting this information yourself with confidence and knowledge. Some patients say they think they can write their own encyclopedia on this disease when they finish their treatment. It's probably true. The majority of biopsies are done simply to remove a small piece of cancerous tissue for diagnosis, which is not part of treatment. This piece of tissue provides information about the type of cancer you have, and gives few specifics about its characteristics. It isn't intended to tell much more than this. The subsequent staging workup will answer the other prognostic questions, so it can be premature to ask the doctor too much about your prognosis, exact stage of disease (beyond what is called clinical staging, not pathology staging), and the precise details of what your treatment will be until your workup has been completed. A routine workup usually includes an imaging study, if one has not been performed, and may include an examination under anesthesia to look at the exact areas involved by the tumor (called the primary site, the site where the tumor started) as well as the rest of the mouth and back of the throat, larynx (voice box), and esophagus to rule out other sites of involvement. This examination is particularly important to do if surgery is being considered as an option for your treatment. Putting together information from your imaging studies along with the biopsy information and exam under anesthesia provides your head and neck surgeon the information needed to determine what your treatment options are.

TYPES OF CANCER

There are a variety of cancer types that can involve the head and neck, and these can vary according to the site involved. Some of the more common tumors encountered are listed below. This list is not meant to be exhaustive as rare tumors can arise from any of the structures of the head and neck.

SQUAMOUS CELL CANCER

Squamous cell cancer is the most common cancer of the head and neck and accounts for 80% of head and neck cancers. It most commonly arises from the lining of the upper aero-digestive tract (mouth, throat, larynx, esophagus) or skin of the head and neck, including the ear or scalp. The majority of squamous cell cancers of the skin are related to sun exposure, while most squamous cell cancers of the upper aero-digestive tract are related to tobacco and alcohol use, although 25% of patients do not have those risk factors. Some patients with a history of human papillomavirus (HPV) infection are at increased risk for squamous cell cancer. Treatment of squamous cell cancer of the head and neck may involve surgery, radiation, or radiation with chemotherapy. Your doctor will make recommendations based on the location involved, the stage of your cancer, and your wishes. Squamous cell carcinoma that involves the oral cavity, bone, or cartilage requires surgery with post-operative radiation. The incidence of spread to lymph nodes in the neck increases with increasing tumor size and needs to be addressed as part of treatment. In addition, certain locations: the upper part of the larynx, the tonsil, and the tongue base are associated with a high incidence of so called "occult" or microscopic cancer in the lymph nodes of greater than 30%, often involving the lymph nodes on *both* sides of the neck, and treatment of these nodes will need to be incorporated into your treatment plan.

ADENOCARCINOMA

Adenocarcinoma most commonly arises in salivary gland tissue or the esophagus, though it can also arise in the sinuses. The prognosis depends on the site involved. When adenocarcinoma arises in the esophagus, the extent of involvement and spread to lymph nodes in the chest will determine whether you are a candidate for surgery or if non-operative therapy is an option. Surgery may involve a thoracic or gastrointestinal surgeon if the cancer arises low in the esophagus, and is followed by post-operative radiation and sometimes chemotherapy. Adenocarcinoma arising from the salivary glands or sinuses on the other hand is usually treated surgically and has a low incidence (10%) of lymph node spread.

SALIVARY GLAND MALIGNANCIES

Salivary gland tissue consists of major salivary glands— the paired parotid glands that fill out our cheeks or the paired sub-mandibular glands just below your jaw line— or minor salivary gland tissue. The minor salivary glands consist of hundreds of tiny glands lining the mouth which cannot be seen with the naked eye; this tissue is also present in small amounts in the throat, larynx, and sinuses. The majority of tumors arising from the parotid glands are benign, while the majority of tumors arising from minor salivary glands are malignant. The most common malignancies are *adenocarcinoma, adenoid cystic carcinoma, mucoepidermoid carcinoma, salivary duct carcinoma*, and a number of rarer tumors. Treatment commonly involves surgery with post-operative radiation based on the pathology. Some tumors such as mucoepidermoid carcinoma and salivary duct carcinoma commonly spread to lymph nodes in the neck, which will require treatment along with the primary tumor. Other tumors such as adenocarcinoma and adenoid cystic carcinoma may spare the lymph nodes. Adenoid cystic carcinoma deserves a special note: This tumor spreads along nerves so surgery to treat this disease is usually aggressive and includes post-operative radiation. Non-operative treatments are usually not successful in achieving a cure for this particular tumor.

SINUS CANCER

The most common sinus cancers are *squamous cell cancer* and *adenocarcinoma*, but a variety of tumors can arise in the sinuses including *esthesioneuroblastoma*, *inverting papilloma*, tumors arising from minor salivary gland tissue such as *adenoid cystic carcinoma* and *mucoepidermoid carcinoma, sarcoma*, and *lymphoma*. With the exception of lymphoma (which is usually treated with chemotherapy, or sometimes radiation), surgery is the mainstay of treatment. Some head and neck surgeons are now able to remove limited sinus tumors endoscopically in highly selected cases.

THYROID CANCER

Thyroid cancer is common, with more than 30,000 people diagnosed per year in the United States. Surgery is the mainstay of treatment for thyroid cancer. The important thing to remember about thyroid cancer is that, in most cases, it is very curable. Prognosis depends on the tumor type and stage. *Papillary* and *follicular* thyroid cancers are sometimes combined under the classification "well-differentiated thyroid cancer" and have a high cure rate.

Treatment involves surgical removal of the thyroid gland with post-operative radioactive iodine if the tumor is larger than 1 cm in size. Sometimes radiation therapy may be recommended for advanced disease. Lymph nodes may need to be removed if these are involved and you will require surveillance to monitor for recurrence, but keep in mind that spread to lymph nodes is very common in this type of cancer (and very curable).

Other types of thyroid cancer include *medullary* thyroid cancer, which may run in families, and *anaplastic* thyroid cancer. These two types are much more aggressive. Medullary thyroid cancer is treated with surgery. Your surgeon may recommend testing family members for the ret-2 protooncogene if you are diagnosed with medullary thyroid cancer. If the test results are positive, family members can undergo thyroid removal to prevent thyroid cancer from occurring. Anaplastic thyroid cancer on the other hand usually progresses very quickly and is not cured with surgery, radiation, or chemotherapy. Your surgeon will talk to you about treatment options.

SKIN CANCER

Skin cancer is one of the most common malignancies and the true incidence is probably unknown, as many small skin cancers may be removed in doctors' offices and not reported to national tumor registries. The most common skin cancers are *basal cell cancer* and *squamous cell cancer*, which are reported with equal frequency, followed by *melanoma*. All of these skin cancers are related to sun exposure. Basal cell cancers are cured by excision, although some basal cell cancers can behave aggressively and require extensive surgery for removal. Radiation is also an option for a small number of basal cell cancers. Squamous cell cancer of the skin can spread to lymph nodes in the parotid gland (a major salivary gland in your cheeks), as well as the lymph nodes in your neck, and should be thoroughly staged before embarking on treatment. Treatment of squamous cell cancer of the skin usually involves surgery and may require post-operative radiation if the tumor shows signs of aggressive behavior on the final pathology report. Melanoma is a less well understood tumor that in early stages can be treated with excision but does carry a risk of spread to lymph nodes in your neck in all but the earliest stages. Your surgeon may recommend a sentinel node biopsy to determine if you need to have all of the lymph nodes from your neck removed.

Merkel cell cancer is a very rare skin cancer and manifests aggressive behavior with a high incidence of spread to other sites in the body. Depending on the location, often a neck dissection (removal of lymph nodes), radiation, and chemotherapy may be recommended.

NASOPHARYNX CANCER

The nasopharynx is the area behind the nasal passages, at the base of the skull. Tumors arising from these areas are uncommon and are seen with increased frequency in certain populations such as people of Chinese descent whose ancestors come from the southern provinces of China or Eskimos. These tumors seem to be related to the Epstein Barr virus (EBV) in many individuals as well as poorly understood genetic factors. Your doctor may want to do a simple blood test to monitor EBV levels before and after treatment. This is not a perfect test, but if EBV levels rise following treatment it can be associated with tumor recurrence. This tumor is very sensitive to radiation and is not usually treated surgically. The majority of cases of nasopharynx cancer are treated non-operatively with radiation therapy and chemotherapy with good results. Surgery is usually reserved for recurrent tumors when additional radiation therapy cannot be given.

LYMPHOMA

Lymphoma is a cancer that arises from lymphoid tissue. It can arise anywhere within the head and neck. This tumor is different from all other tumor types previously described because the treatment is always medical, not surgical. However, a surgical biopsy may be required to provide the pathologist with sufficient tissue to make the diagnosis as well as test for certain tumor markers, but treatment consists of chemotherapy and sometimes radiation therapy, depending on the type of lymphoma.

UNKNOWN PRIMARY CANCER

An unknown primary tumor is one that is first detected in an enlarged lymph node, meaning the tumor has already spread to lymph nodes, but the primary site where the tumor started may not be readily apparent. The majority (90%) of unknown primary tumors are squamous cell cancers arising from somewhere in the head and neck. Often times the primary site can be found during a thorough head and neck examination, but many times these have remained microscopic despite spreading to lymph nodes.

In 10% of cases, the tumor arises from somewhere in the lung or abdomen. Finding the primary site is critical. Otherwise all of the likely sites where the primary tumor might be hiding need to be treated with radiation, which means giving radiation from the nasopharynx (behind the nose) all the way down to the start of the upper esophagus. Your surgeon will want to perform an examination under anesthesia and biopsy the most likely sites, which include the base of the tongue and the tonsils. Because many unknown primary tumors arise from the tonsil, tonsillectomy is performed to allow the pathologists to look for microscopic tumors hidden in the tonsils in this scenario. In some cases, the primary site is never found. It is thought that possibly the immune system has kept such tumors from growing larger,—though not from spreading to lymph nodes. While this is a good sign, treatment still has to be directed at all the "likely suspects" in order to cure the cancer.

SARCOMA

Sarcomas are rare tumors that can arise anywhere within the head and neck. They can be associated with a history of radiation exposure. Because these tumors are rare, treatment really needs to be performed at a major cancer center that sees enough of these cases to have real experience. Large centers will often have sarcoma experts. The treatment of sarcoma is surgical with wide margins, but wide margins are often not possible in the head and neck. As a result, tumor recurrence rates are high, and chemotherapy and radiation are used as adjuncts to surgery. An exception is rhabdomyosarcoma, which is seen predominantly in younger patients and children, and is usually highly sensitive to chemotherapy and radiation.

PARAGANGLIOMAS

These are rare tumors that arise from nerves in the neck or at the base of the skull or from the carotid artery. They run in families in 10% of cases, and if there is a family history, other family members should get checked as well. Surgery is the mainstay of therapy, as these tumors are not sensitive to radiation or chemotherapy. However, much of the discussion that follows in this book, with the exception of tumor staging, applies to patients with paragangliomas, as surgery can affect speech and swallowing function depending on how big the tumor is and where it is located.

TUMOR GRADE

The grade of the tumor cells may also be recorded as part of the pathology report and is a measure of how abnormal the cancer cells look under the microscope. Grades are well-differentiated, moderately differentiated, or poorly differentiated; some pathologists assign the numbers 1, 2, or 3 to refer to grade or simply say "low grade" (grades 1 and 2) or "high grade" (grade 3). Some pathologists use the term "intermediate grade" to refer to grade 2 tumors. These tumors often have features that make them more of a low-grade or high-grade tumor.

- Grade 1: slow growing and might also be referred to as "well differentiated" cells

- Grade 2: average growing and may be called "moderately differentiated cells"

- Grade 3: rapidly growing and may be termed "poorly differentiated cells"

Don't be surprised—or alarmed—if your report says grade 3. This doesn't mean that cells are growing extraordinarily fast and you have an emergency on your hands. This is a relative, descriptive term, and grade is not the same thing as stage.

Your doctor may wish to have the pathologist test a biopsy specimen for the human papillomavirus (HPV). There is a known link between the HPV virus and squamous cell cancer of the tongue base or tonsil, and knowledge of HPV status in patients with tonsil and tongue base cancer has prognostic value.

UNDERSTANDING CANCER STAGE

Stage and grade are often confused, and not surprisingly as the staging system is confusing initially. Grade, as we just discussed, is related to cell growth and really does not provide much information in the way of prognostic value except for certain tumors like mucoepidermoid cancer, where grade can be associated with stage. Stage is the most important variable and combines several pieces of information (the size of the tumor, nodal involvement, and other organ involvement) and is used to provide survival estimates. Remember, however, that you are not a statistic. You are an individual person whose cure rate is either going to be all or none. People fall on both sides of the statistics to produce these numbers. You are not a number!

The TNM stage (Tumor, Nodes, Metastases) is used to come up with an overall stage based on the size of the primary tumor, the degree of lymph node involvement in your neck, and the presence or absence of distant metastases (spread beyond the head and neck region). For most tumors of the head and neck, the stage is determined based on the factors listed in Tables 1-1, 1-2, and 1-3. The staging system is different for esophageal cancer, nasopharyngeal cancer, thyroid cancer, and lymphoma. In addition, some very rare tumors such as sarcoma have their own staging systems based on the pathological subtype and are beyond the scope of this book.

STAGING EXPLAINED

The most common staging system is the American Joint Commission on Cancer (AJCC) system which uses the tumor stage (T stage, **Table 1-1**), nodal stage (N stage, **Table 1-2**), and presence of distant metastases (M stage) to come up with a combined score (**Table 1-3**). This overall "TNM" stage is what is usually referred to when people speak of cancer stage and has the most prognostic value in terms of survival; it will be the staging system referred to in the remaining chapters of this book. Accurate staging usually requires an imaging study for advanced stage tumors. Imaging can help the surgeon see how far the cancer has spread locally and what structures are involved. In addition, there are certain radiologic criteria used to determine if lymph nodes look suspicious for involvement or not— even when they cannot be palpated by the surgeon. Your stage may change after an imaging study.

The simplified staging system explained on the next page applies to most tumors of the head and neck involving the upper aero-digestive tract (sinus, nasal cavity, oral cavity, oropharynx, larynx, hypopharynx) with the exception of nasopharynx, thyroid, and esophageal cancer as well as melanoma and lymphoma, which all have their own staging systems.

Stage o is noninvasive cancer, or CIS (*carcinoma in situ*). In this case, the cancer cells are limited to the superficial layers of the skin or mucosa and have not invaded the basement membrane separating the superficial tissues from the deep tissues. The size of the tumor in this case does not

---

TABLE 1-1. PRIMARY TUMOR STAGING FOR HEAD AND NECK CANCER

To = the primary tumor cannot be found (unknown primary)

T1 = tumor less than 2 cm (1″)

T2 = tumor greater than 2 cm but less than 4 cm (2″)

T3 = tumor greater than 4 cm, or tumor involving a vocal cord causing paralysis or with limited spread beyond the larynx, or involving the bone of the sinuses for sinus and nasopharynx tumors

T4 = tumor that has spread beyond the site of origin to involve nearby structures such as bone or muscle

---

TABLE 1-2. LYMPH NODE STAGING FOR HEAD AND NECK CANCER

No = no obvious lymph node involvement

N1 = a single enlarged lymph node, less than 3 cm in size, on the same side as the primary tumor

N2 = a single enlarged lymph node, greater than 3 cm in size but less than 6 cm in size, or more than one lymph node involved that is less than 6 cm in size

    N2A: a single lymph node on the same side as the tumor between 3 cm and 6 cm

    N2B: more than one lymph node, on the same side as the tumor, less than 6 cm

    N2C: lymph nodes involved on both sides of the neck, or the opposite side of the neck from the tumor, less than 6 cm in size.

N3 = an enlarged lymph node that is 6 cm or larger

---

need to be measured to determine the stage. It is the lack of invasion that is important. There is no lymph node spread in such cases, as the tumor has not invaded deeply enough to reach lymphatic vessels. Removal is curative!

Stage 1 cancer is invasive cancer with a tumor diameter less than 2 cm (less than 1″) or involving only one area of the larynx or sinuses; this is called a T1 tumor. Stage 1 cancer means there is no evidence of cancer in the lymph nodes.

Stage 2 cancer is a larger cancer with a tumor diameter is between 2 cm and 4 cm (1″ to 2″), or in the case of larynx or sinus cancer, involving more than one site: this is called a T2 tumor. Stage 2 cancer means there is no evidence of cancer within the lymph nodes.

Stage 3 cancer can have a few different scenarios as shown in Table 1-1. This can be a tumor that is larger than 4 cm (2″), involves a vocal cord, or involves the bone of the sinuses or nasal cavity. This is called a T3 tumor. Lymph node involvement affects stage in this case. A cancer is considered stage 3 if one has a T3 tumor with no lymph nodes involved or limited node involvement (N1), or any T1, T2, or T3 tumor with limited lymph node involvement (N1).

Stage 4 cancer refers to one of three possible scenarios. A large primary tumor that has spread outside of the site of origin to involve nearby structures, such as bone or muscle, is considered a T4 tumor, and is stage 4 cancer, regardless of whether or not lymph nodes are involved. The extent of involvement of surrounding tissues is important in determining whether or not surgery can be performed safely. In addition, any patient with "bulky" node disease—a lymph node that is larger than 3 cm or multiple lymph nodes involved in the neck—is considered stage 4.

Finally the presence of distant metastases (spread beyond the head and neck, to involve the lungs, liver, or bone, among other sites), places one in the category of stage 4 cancer. This particular situation—when the tumor has already spread throughout the body—is a contraindication to surgery, as surgery does not address these other distant sites that are involved, and non-operative therapy is used. The presence of distant metastases is associated with poorer survival. It is important to rule out a second tumor, such as a new lung cancer, before assuming that a lung lesion is a distant metastasis, which may require a biopsy.

- Early stage cancers are considered stages 0, 1, and 2.

- The presence of lymph node involvement automatically bumps up the stage to stage 3 or 4.

- Advanced stage cancers are considered stages 3 and 4.

- All patients with distant metastases (spread of cancer to lung, liver, bone, brain, kidney, etc.) are considered stage 4 (but not all stage 4 cancers have distant metastases).

These stages can be modified for specific organ sites. For example, staging of sinus or nasopharynx tumors takes into account what structures surrounding the sinuses are involved (or not). Nasopharynx cancer has its own special staging system because lymph node involvement is so common in this disease and does not have the same implications that it does for other tumors of the head and neck.

TABLE 1-3. OVERALL TUMOR STAGE (THE TNM CLASSIFICATION) FOR HEAD AND NECK CANCERS

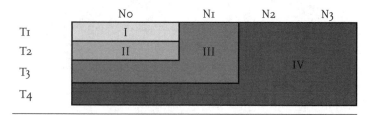

	N0	N1	N2	N3
T1	I			
T2	II	III		
T3			IV	
T4				

Cancer of the esophagus has its own staging system based on the depth of tumor involvement through the wall of the esophagus. An early-stage tumor is one that is confined to the lining of the esophagus, while advanced-stage tumors involve not only the lining but the muscular wall of the esophagus. Involvement of lymph nodes, in this case lymph nodes in the chest, similarly alters staging, with lymph node involvement resulting in a more advanced-stage cancer.

MELANOMA

Melanoma has its own staging system and is staged based on the depth of invasion of skin structures (see Table 1-4 and Table 1-5). Your surgeon may mention the Clark system or the Breslow system. In both staging systems the depth of invasion is used to describe the primary (skin) tumor. Breslow thickness of invasion has replaced the Clark level as the more accurate method of measuring tumor penetration. Measurement of tumor thickness requires complete excision of the primary melanoma tumor to determine the exact stage, not just a biopsy. The presence or absence of ulceration of the surface of the tumor is an important prognostic sign that influences staging. Node staging is based on number of lymph nodes or the presence of satellite metastases—small deposits of tumor surrounding the primary tumor that are not continuous, or part of, the primary tumor. Metastases are staged as either absent (M0) or present (M1).

The overall TNM stage for melanoma is based on tumor thickness, lymph node metastases, and distant metastases (See **Table 1-6**). Stage 1 and Stage 2 melanoma is melanoma with no evidence of node involvement or distant metastases. Stage 3 melanoma is melanoma with lymph node metastases but no distant metastases. Stage 4 melanoma is any melanoma with distant metastases.

TABLE 1-4. MELANOMA PRIMARY TUMOR STAGE

T1 = tumor thickness less than or equal to 1 mm
    A: without ulceration
    B: with ulceration

T2 = tumor thickness greater than 1 mm but less than 2 mm
    A: without ulceration
    B: with ulceration

T3 = tumor thickness greater than 2 mm but less than or equal to 4 mm
    A: without ulceration
    B: with ulceration

T4 = tumor thickness greater than 4 mm
    A: without ulceration
    B: with ulceration

TABLE 1-5. MELANOMA LYMPH NODE STAGE

N0 = no lymph node involvement

N1 = a single involved lymph node

N2 = 2 to 3 lymph nodes involved

N3 = 4 or more lymph nodes involved or satellite metastases: areas of visible tumor growth extending beyond the primary melanoma which suggest spread along lymphatic drainage pathways

---

TABLE 1-6. MELANOMA TNM STAGE

Stage 1 = T1, or T2 without ulceration: no nodes or distant metastases

Stage 2 = T2 with ulceration, any T3 or T4: no nodes or distant metastases

Stage 3 = any T stage with nodal metastases but no distant metastases

Stage 4 = any T or N stage with distant metastases

THYROID CANCER

Thyroid cancer has its own staging classification, which is based on size and lymph node involvement (see **Table 1-7**). The primary tumor size is important and is measured similar to the AJCC staging system described above for head and neck tumors. Lymph nodes are described as either not involved (N0) or involved (N1). Distant metastases are considered either absent (M0) or present (M1). Thyroid cancer staging systems differ based on tumor type. There is a separate staging system for papillary and follicular thyroid cancer that includes age of 45 years or greater as a prognostic variable. All anaplastic thyroid cancers are automatically staged as stage 4 cancer.

There are only 2 stages for papillary or follicular thyroid cancer for patients under 45 years of age, who are considered to have a more favorable prognosis: This is based on the absence (stage 1) or presence (stage 2) of distant metastases (see **Table 1-7**).

TABLE 1-7. PAPILLARY AND FOLLICULAR THYROID CANCER STAGING FOR PATIENTS UNDER 45 YEARS OF AGE

	M0	M1
Any T, any N	I	II

TABLE 1-8. PAPILLARY AND FOLLICULAR THYROID CANCER STAGING FOR PATIENTS 45 YEARS OF AGE OR OLDER AND FOR MEDULLARY THYROID CANCER REGARDLESS OF AGE

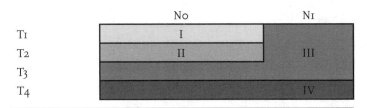

	N0	N1
T1	I	
T2	II	III
T3		
T4		IV

There are four stages of papillary or follicular thyroid cancer for patients 45 years of age or older (see Table 1-8). The presence of distant metastases in patients 45 years or older automatically makes a papillary or follicular thyroid cancer stage 4.

The staging system for medullary thyroid carcinoma is similar to the staging system used for papillary and follicular thyroid cancer in patients who are 45 years of age or greater—with the exception that age does not factor into the staging of medullary thyroid cancer.

THE DIFFERENCE BETWEEN CLINICAL AND PATHOLOGICAL STAGING

There is a difference between clinical staging and pathologic staging. Clinical staging is based on clinical examination findings, including imaging studies. Pathologic staging is based on what the pathologist actually sees following surgical removal of the tumor and lymph nodes. Sometimes lymph nodes that appear normal may contain microscopic cancer, and so the pathologic stage would be different from the clinical stage, and vice versa. Similarly, sometimes involvement of bone and muscle can only be determined or ruled out by the pathologist's microscope, and this can result in a difference between the clinical and pathological stage as well. It is important to remember that if you read the literature on your particular type of cancer, the stage that is used in the majority of publications refers to the clinical stage, not the pathological stage. This is because all patients have a clinical stage assigned to them, while not all patients undergo surgery and therefore not all patients have a known pathological stage. So data regarding survival and cure rates are based on the clinical stage. But sometimes the pathologic stage information is used to determine the need for radiation or chemotherapy after surgery, particularly in cases of nerve involvement or lymph node involvement not suspected preoperatively.

THE BOTTOM LINE: TALK TO YOUR DOCTOR

The discussion in this chapter is not meant to be all-inclusive but to serve as an introduction to head and neck cancer staging. Be sure to talk to your head and neck surgeon about your specific situation. It is our hope that a better understanding of what stage means will help you to have these discussions.

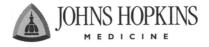

CHAPTER 2

My Team—Meeting Your Treatment Team

Erin J. Blume, BS, RHIA
Carol S. Maragos, MSN, CRNP, CNOR

There will be many people on your oncology team helping you through treatment. Each has a specific role and specialty related to head and neck cancer and its treatment. Below is a list of the major team players.

- Surgical oncologist. Otolaryngologist (ear nose and throat doctor) who specializes in head and neck cancer and performs head and neck surgery. This is usually the first doctor you see when you are newly diagnosed or seeking diagnosis.

- Medical oncologist. Specially trained doctor who uses chemotherapy to destroy cancer cells.

- Radiation oncologist. Specially trained doctor who uses radiation therapy, a treatment that uses high doses of radiation, to kill cancer cells and stop them from spreading.

- Radiologist. A specially trained doctor who reads the scans, X-rays, and other images such as CT, MRI or PET scans that are done to stage and follow your cancer.

- Plastic surgeon. Specialist who performs reconstruction to preserve or restore both the appearance and function of the involved area.

- Prosthodontist. Dentist who specializes in the restoration of oral function by creating prostheses and restorations (i.e., complete dentures, crowns, implant retained/supported restorations).

- Pathologist. A behind the scenes specialist who looks under the microscope at your biopsy tissue to determine the type and size of tumor and provides important prognostic information, which is used to determine your treatment plan.

- Residents, interns, and nurse practitioners. Under the direction of your surgeon, they may assist in the operating room and manage your post-operative care.

- Nurses. You will meet several nurses who will help you through your treatment as they are located in every department involved in your care. Some of the functions they perform include patient education, assessing your clinical needs, providing your care after surgery, administering chemotherapy drugs, and evaluating your progress during radiation and chemotherapy.

- Speech Language Pathologist (SLP). A licensed professional who assesses, diagnoses, treats, and helps to prevent disorders related to speech, language, voice, and swallowing.

- Social worker. This person helps arrange for any personal needs you may have from assisting with financial issues, arranging home health care (if necessary), to providing social networks.

- Clinical Coordinator/Patient Navigator. This relatively new breed of health care worker helps you navigate the system so you can receive your treatment in a timely manner. They help coordinate your care and refer you to the appropriate services you need.

- Dietician. A health care provider who makes recommendations for proper nutrition.

- Home care coordinator. A nurse who orders supplies and equipment for home and who sets up home nursing care.

MAKING YOUR INITIAL APPOINTMENT

The doctor you meet with for your first consultation should be a head and neck surgical oncologist. This is a doctor who specializes in the field of cancer surgery and, within that specialty, head and neck cancer. If the cancer center or hospital where you are going has a web site, you should look at it to view faculty biographies and learn whether there is a particular doctor that you think you'd prefer to see over another. When you select this specialist, research his or her credentials, board certification, the volume of head and neck cancer patients he or she treats as well as how many head and neck cancer patients are treated annually at the institution.

Most facilities arrange for patient appointments quite promptly. It is not an emergency to be seen in the next day or two, though you may feel like it is. When calling to make an appointment, please have the following information available:

- Personal contact information (phone numbers, address, etc.)

- Diagnosis

- Details of diagnosis (tests performed, biopsy results, etc.)

- Specific information about any treatment received

- Names and phone numbers of all physicians who have provided care related to diagnosis, including primary care provider

- Insurance information, including any necessary HMO authorization

When you contact the facility for an appointment, be sure to get the specific address, directions, and what time you are to report there. If you haven't been to this facility before, allow yourself time to find it, park, and get to the location where the doctor will be. Being late will only stress you more.

WHAT TO BRING WITH YOU FOR THAT FIRST CONSULTATION

The scheduler you speak with should also provide you with instructions regarding what to bring. Just in case the information isn't clear, below is some information to help ensure that your visit is as productive and efficient as possible for you and the doctor who will be seeing you.

Most physicians require that certain medical information is forwarded in advance of the appointment or brought on the day of the appointment. This information may include:

- Outside scans and reports (for example, CT, MRI, or PET scans).

- Pathology slides and reports.

- Medical records pertinent to diagnosis and care (surgical reports, treatment summary, etc.), including specific information about surgeries you've had as well as any chemotherapy and radiation treatment. Specific treatment records describing chemotherapy drugs utilized or amount of radiation therapy treatment are extremely helpful.

WHAT ELSE TO BRING FOR THIS INITIAL VISIT

Bring a detailed list of medications you are currently taking, including vitamins and herbs, what allergies you may have, and your family history for cancers, heart disease, diabetes, lung disease, and other serious illnesses. It is important for your medical summary and may influence some decision making about your treatment recommendations.

WHO TO BRING WITH YOU TO THE FIRST CONSULTATIVE VISIT

Bring a trusted family member or friend with you. When people are stressed they only hear and retain 10 percent of what is said to them. The doctor will provide you with a lot of information about your diagnosis, treatment options, and side effects. You may not be able to process it all or you may feel overwhelmed by the information. The person with you serves as a second set of ears and can take notes so you can review it again later after you've had time to process the information you've been given.

WHAT QUESTIONS TO ASK DURING YOUR VISIT

Having a list of questions prepared in advance is helpful in making the time you have with the doctor as efficient and optimal as possible. Below is a list to help you get started.

Treatment

1. What are your personal and the center's experience with this specific type/location of cancer?

2. Are there different types of this cancer? If so, what type do I have and what's the significance?

3. What stage is the cancer? Has it spread? If it has not spread, does that mean it won't? If it has spread, where is it?

4. What is the time window for treatments to maximize a good prognosis?

5. What are the treatment plan options that are being considered? What are the advantages and disadvantages of each treatment plan option? Which do you recommend for me and why?

6. What are the treatment's side effects?

7. What other information is needed and what tests need to be completed before initiating the actual treatment?

8. How long will treatment last?

   a. Is the surgery done as an "in-patient" in the hospital? How soon would it be scheduled? How long might I have to stay in the hospital? What can I expect the day(s) after surgery? What type of home care might I need? Does someone need to stay with me when I'm at home? Will my life be changed in any way?

   b. When would radiation treatment (and/or chemotherapy) begin, and what is the frequency/ duration for that phase? If a multi-day course of radiation or chemotherapy is planned, do I stay in the hospital? If I am released to home, in what condition will I be after radiation or chemotherapy? What level of care will be required at home?

9. Are there any clinical studies being conducted or is other information available about my type of cancer that may help me understand and mange my condition?

Quality of Life

10. I question my strength of character to get through this. What can I do to help myself?

11. What issues will I need to deal with as part of the post-op recovery, and what resources will I have available to me?

12. What issues will I need to deal with as part of radiation/chemotherapy and recovery?

13. What other issues will I need to deal with?

14. What can I do to deal with my mental anguish, fragile emotional state, and anxiety associated with all of this?

15. What kind of activity level can I expect to have at home and at work?

16. Do you have a support group for head and neck cancer patients?

17. May I speak to a head and neck cancer survivor volunteer who has had a similar treatment plan?

After Treatment

18. How will my normal activities be affected long term?

19. Will I be able to return to work (after recovery) and communicate effectively?

20. From a prevention standpoint, what was the likely cause(s) of this cancer, and what can I do to prevent its reoccurrence?

21. What can I do personally to increase my chances of success during treatment and beyond?

22. What level of therapy do you require so that I can regain my effective speech and swallowing?

23. How long might I expect to be in speech or swallowing therapy?

24. Who will be my contact here for questions that I may have?

25. When my treatment is complete, what will the follow-up schedule be?

WHAT TESTS NEED TO BE DONE

After reviewing your scans, the physician may decide he or she wants additional imaging done to provide more detail about where the cancer is located. Don't be surprised or caught off guard by this possibility. You want your physician to be thorough.

HOW TO BEST CONTACT TEAM MEMBERS

Request business cards from each health care provider you see and ask what the office procedure is for responding to questions and concerns you may have. Usually there is one contact person on your team who is designated to address questions, who you can rely on to serve in this role. Also determine if you can communicate with any of the team by email. When communicating with your health care team, be succinct and thoughtful.

NAVIGATING APPOINTMENTS

Some cancer centers have patient navigators. When you inquire about whether your cancer center has such a resource, find out about the process for assisting you with appointment scheduling, getting test results, getting scheduled for your surgery, and seeing a medical oncologist and radiation oncologist. It's also a good idea to find out the availability of someone for general support, especially to address any other clinical needs that may arise.

FINANCIAL IMPLICATIONS OF TREATMENT AND INSURANCE CLEARANCE

There is no convenient time to get this disease; the diagnosis alone can create havoc in your life. If you are working outside the home, you will be taking time off for your surgery and possibly for other treatment afterward. Getting everything squared away early is smart. Finding out how much sick leave you have, short-term disability coverage, co-payment information, prescription coverage, and other medical expense issues is helpful for planning your budget. Your insurance company may require referrals to be obtained in order to see certain specialists, get tests done, get surgery authorized, as well as other treatments. If you need help with these things, ask for a social worker to assist you. Cancer centers also have financial assistants for this purpose.

There may be some recommended treatments relating to clinical trials. Some treatments may be covered by your insurance and others may not. If participating in a clinical trial, obtain a copy of the informed consent so you're aware what the trial will and will not cover.

If you lack health insurance, there are resources available for people who need help and meet certain criteria for financial assistance and coverage of their cancer treatment expenses. Some states even have special grants for residents precisely for this purpose. Check with the social worker at the facility where you are being treated to get assistance and referrals. There are also organizations that provide support for transportation to and from treatment visits, provide food for you and your family, and even assist with medication coverage. These resources aren't available in every state so rely on the social worker to tell you more about what is available for your geographic area. Be proactive in asking to meet with the social worker to discuss what support services are available for you as well.

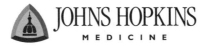

CHAPTER 3

TAKING ACTION—
COMPREHENSIVE TREATMENT
CONSIDERATIONS

Christine G. Gourin, MD FACS

This chapter will describe each phase of treatment and the decision making involved to determine whether you need that treatment or not. Head and neck cancer treatment can include surgery, chemotherapy, and radiation therapy alone or in combination. Whether or not you will need one, two, or all of these therapies depends on the stage and sites involved by your cancer. Let's review each one.

SURGICAL TREATMENT

Surgery for head and neck cancer is a terrifying prospect for many patients. Most of us face any type of surgery with some dread, and the fear that surgery may change one's physical appearance, speech, or ability to swallow causes many patients to try to avoid surgery whenever possible. While it is true that surgery for head and neck cancer may involve some change in your appearance or function, the degree to which this may happen depends on where your cancer is located and how advanced it is. In some cases surgery offers the best chance for cure, and you should talk through all of your concerns and options with your surgeon. These discussions are critical and should take place before surgery.

Surgery is the preferred therapy for patients with tumors of the oral cavity regardless of stage, patients with salivary gland and thyroid cancer, and for most patients with early-stage disease without evidence of metastases for other sites of the head and neck. The type of surgery required depends on the primary site of the tumor. For oral cavity tumors, surgery can range from removal of a small part of the oral cavity to more extensive surgery requiring removal of part of the jaw. Post-operative radiation is used for aggressive tumors such as those tumors that are stage 3 or 4 or tumors with signs of extracapsular spread of tumor in lymph nodes or perineural invasion (spread along nerves). Chemotherapy may be added to post-operative radiation for tumors with extracapsular spread, as there is some literature that suggests a small survival advantage with the addition of chemotherapy in this circumstance, however, this decision requires discussion with your doctor before proceeding as the benefits remain controversial.

Patients with salivary gland or thyroid cancers require surgery for removal, with post-operative radiation used for tumors that have aggressive histologic patterns identified by the pathologist on examination of the specimen. Well-differentiated thyroid cancers, such as papillary cancer, may require additional treatment with radioactive iodine based on the size and stage of the tumor. Radioactive iodine is not the same thing as traditional radiation therapy but is a so-called biological treatment in which radioactive iodine is taken orally by the patient and is taken up by any remaining microscopic thyroid tissue, which absorbs iodine and is then killed by the radioactivity incorporated into the iodine itself.

EARLY-STAGE DISEASE

Patients with early stage tumors (stage 1 or 2) of other sites, such as the oral cavity, oropharynx, or larynx can be treated with surgery alone, and in this situation surgery is often preferable to non-surgical treatment such as radiation. When tumors are detected at an early stage, the surgery is often a limited procedure, such as removing part of the vocal cord for early-stage larynx cancer, or the tonsil and the effects of surgery are often limited and easily adapted to with few sequelae. The advantage to surgery in this situation is that radiation therapy can often be avoided altogether. Radiation has side effects that are permanent, such as tissue fibrosis (stiffening) that can impact swallowing, dry mouth (xerostomia) which is permanent, and once radiation therapy has been used to treat an area, radiation usually cannot be used again in tissue that has been treated with radiation with a reasonable chance of cure. The surgery required to treat a recurrence is often a more advanced and extensive operation, as surgical margins to determine if the tumor has been completely removed are difficult to assess in radiated tissue. So radiation to "save" the larynx, for example, in the case of early-stage larynx cancer, can result in loss of the entire larynx if the cancer recurs or a new tumor develops. For oral cavity tumors, radiation is rarely indicated as primary treatment, as the failure rate and side effects are high compared with surgery.

When surgery can be used for early-stage cancers, it is preferable to radiation therapy to keep this in reserve for the future, like an insurance policy. If the surgical specimen shows aggressive features on pathology such as perineural invasion, your surgeon may recommend post-operative radiation to improve the chances of cure. Radiation in this circumstance is used at a lower dose than when it is used "up-front" to treat cancer, thus lowering the incidence of severe swallowing-related side effects.

Chemotherapy or chemoradiation (chemotherapy plus radiation given together) are never indicated for early-stage disease because there is no data to support the use of chemotherapy for early-stage disease; it is just too much treatment.

ADVANCED-STAGE DISEASE

Patients with advanced-stage tumors (stage 3 or 4 cancer) require what is called "multimodality therapy": that is, more than one type of treatment. When surgery is used to remove advanced-stage tumors, it is followed by radiation therapy or chemoradiation, depending on the pathology report. We know from years of experience that the failure rate of single modality therapy, such as surgery alone, is much greater than when surgery is combined with post-operative radiation therapy. Surgery followed by post-operative radiation remains the recommended initial treatment for patients with advanced oral cavity tumors. Again, for oral cavity tumors, there is no good data to support the use of chemoradiation as initial treatment. Surgery is known to result in improved survival and function (swallowing, voice) in patients with the most advanced stage larynx or hypopharynx tumors, as well as most skin cancers and salivary gland tumors. Patients with stage 3 larynx cancer may have the option of larynx preservation surgery, which preserves part of the larynx, or chemoradiation. Both treatment options have equivalent survival rates.

For oropharyngeal tumors, surgery should be discussed with your surgeon carefully because data suggests that radiation or chemoradiation as initial treatment is equivalent to surgery followed by radiation. Because surgery of the oropharynx can often result in significant functional impairment from removal of muscles used for speech and swallowing, the decision to pursue surgery for advanced-stage oropharyngeal cancer should only be made after careful consideration. Because patients with advanced-stage oropharyngeal cancer often have advanced lymph node involvement and often require chemoradiation, it is reasonable to pursue chemoradiation initially in this circumstance, realizing that chemoradiation carries its own risk of potential functional impairment.

When more than one treatment choice is possible, you must educate yourself about the side effects to be anticipated from all treatment options so you can make an educated decision. It may be helpful to talk to patients who have gone through treatment for similar tumors; your doctor or local support group can put you in contact with survivors. Such discussions can be very enlightening and useful.

SURGERY FOR RECURRENT DISEASE AFTER RADIATION THERAPY OR CHEMORADIATION

Patients who develop a recurrence of their tumor following initial treatment with radiation therapy or chemoradiation can no longer receive those modalities to treat the recurrence with the intent to cure. These patients usually face surgery. In some circumstances, re-irradiation can be performed. However, in that case the dose of radiation that can be used is often limited by the amount previously given. There is a limit to how much radiation can be given to tissue without causing normal tissue to die. Re-irradiation is rarely curative because curative doses cannot be safely given, and often the tumor is not radiation sensitive because it recurred despite radiation. One major exception is nasopharyngeal cancer, which can often be treated successfully with re-irradiation for recurrence. Most patients with recurrence following radiation or chemoradiation are not able to receive additional radiation and will require surgery for "salvage" in an attempt to cure the tumor when it can be removed, as long as there is no evidence of distant metastatic disease beyond the head and neck area. Free flap reconstruction is often required, because tissue healing after radiation is poor, and the use of tissue from other parts of the body that have not received radiation can improve wound healing and outcomes. This is discussed in greater detail in the section on reconstruction.

NECK DISSECTION

Neck dissection is a term for lymph node removal. In head and neck cancer, the primary site is the area where the tumor originates and when these tumors spread to lymph nodes, the lymph nodes in the neck, also called cervical lymph nodes, are the first areas that cancers may drain to. Some patients may present with an enlarged cervical lymph node, which may be the first sign of head and neck cancer. When patients with head and neck cancer have enlarged lymph nodes that can be palpated on examination, we say they have "node-positive" disease. As discussed in Chapter 1, this automatically makes the cancer a stage 3 or 4, depending on how large the lymph nodes are. Some patients have no evidence of enlarged lymph nodes on examination ("node-negative" disease), but we know from the experience of thousands of patients who have gone before that certain primary tumors have a high incidence of microscopic cancer in the lymph nodes. This can be unilateral (one-sided) or bilateral (both sides of the neck), depending on the primary site the tumor arose from. Therefore, even though your neck may feel normal, your surgeon may recommend a lymph node dissection of one or both sides of the neck. If your risk of having cancer in the cervical lymph nodes is greater than 15% to 20%, then treatment of cancer must include treatment of the neck.

If you are undergoing surgery to remove the primary tumor, removal of the cervical lymph nodes is recommended if you have enlarged lymph nodes or have a risk of microscopic lymph node involvement that is greater than 15% to 20%. Not all enlarged lymph nodes contain cancer; conversely, not all normal lymph nodes are cancer-free. If surgery to treat your cancer has been recommended by your doctor, in all but the earliest stage cancers this will involve some type of neck dissection.

Neck dissection to treat node-negative disease—a neck without evidence of enlarged lymph nodes—is usually called a selective neck dissection. Your surgeon will remove just those node levels that are most likely to carry cancer. Which areas these are depends on the tumor primary site. In the old days, patients used to undergo radical neck dissection—removal of all lymph nodes as well as the sternocleidomastoid muscle, accessory nerve, and jugular vein, regardless of where the tumor was located because knowledge of tumor drainage patterns to lymph nodes was not known. Based on those years, we now know which lymph node levels are most likely involved, as tumors tend to drain in predictable ways based on the site of origin and such extensive neck dissection can be avoided in patients who don't have enlarged lymph nodes on examination.

More extensive neck dissection that removes nodes from all areas of the neck is performed for patients with enlarged lymph nodes at the time of their cancer diagnosis. This can be termed a "comprehensive neck dissection," meaning all five nodal levels are removed, or a "modified radical neck dissection," which refers to a comprehensive neck dissection with removal of the sternocleidomastoid muscle, accessory nerve, or jugular vein. These structures and this type of neck dissection are discussed in more detail in Chapter 4.

SENTINEL NODE BIOPSY

In selected cases, your surgeon may recommend a sentinel node biopsy to determine if cancer has spread to lymph nodes or not. This is commonly used for patients with breast cancer, for example, but has very limited use in the head and neck so far. The reason is that we just don't know whether or not sentinel node biopsy can accurately determine the status of the lymph nodes in the head and neck for most types of head and neck cancer. A sentinel node is the first node that a cancer drains to. The surgeon identifies which node is the sentinel node by injecting a radiolabelled isotope or tracer into the tumor and then getting a nuclear medicine scan to see which nodes take up the tracer. Just because a node takes up the tracer does not mean that the node contains cancer. It means that it is the sentinel node or first node to receive drainage from the tumor site. The surgeon then uses a gamma camera that can measure radioactivity emitted by this node to identify the sentinel node and remove it to see if cancer cells are present or not. Because this is only used for cases without evidence of node spread (node-negative patients), the pathologist cannot determine if microscopic cells are present on a frozen section, which can miss small cells, and instead needs at least several days to look through the entire specimen. When cancer cells are found in a sentinel node, a neck dissection is needed, which is usually performed at a second operation after the pathology evaluation is completed. The advantage to sentinel node biopsy is that if no cancer is found in the sentinel node, neck dissection can be avoided.

Sentinel node biopsy is used commonly for melanomas of the skin, where it has been shown to be highly predictive of lymph node spread. In other tumors of the head and neck, its use is limited, and it is not an accepted standard of care yet. The primary tumor has to be accessible to being injected with the tracer by a radiologist. Skin tumors are easily accessible; most other head and neck sites are not. Currently sentinel node biopsy is being studied in clinical trials of patients with squamous cell cancer of the oral cavity. Preliminary studies show that the head and neck usually has multiple sentinel nodes, and in half of all cases in whom cancer is found in a sentinel node, more than one sentinel node is positive for cancer. Removal of multiple sentinel nodes can in such cases be similar to performing a selective neck dissection, which gives more prognostic information and may be therapeutic. As of this writing, for head and neck tumors, sentinel node biopsy is only appropriate for melanomas of the skin of the head and neck.

RECONSTRUCTION

Depending on the size and location of your primary tumor, your surgeon may recommend reconstruction with a graft or flap to improve the functional outcome and appearance after surgery. In general, the simplest reconstructive option that will achieve a good result is used. Many areas can undergo "primary closure" where the surrounding tissue can be closed over the defect. When there is not enough tissue to close the area, in cases like skin cancer, small areas can be left open to close spontaneously through new tissue from the edges growing in. This is called "secondary closure," and an example would be the way an abrasion or skinned knee will heal through scarring. Local skin flaps can be used to close larger defects of the skin after removal of skin or parotid cancer. These take advantage of the loose skin of the neck or areas of the face that can be moved into the defect through carefully planned incisions to make the end result cosmetically appealing. Larger defects require the use of tissue from other parts of the body.

For patients undergoing reconstruction it is important to look as the surgical site as a work in progress. Reconstruction takes weeks to months to take shape and also may require additional surgery for the final result to be achieved. Do not allow yourself to get discouraged!

Skin grafts

Skin grafts are commonly used to close small defects of the nose, scalp, oral cavity, and oropharynx. Skin grafts are thin sheets of skin and are usually "split thickness," meaning the upper half of the skin layer is removed, leaving some skin in place that will heal over. These are harvested most commonly from the upper thigh and placed over the defect and sewn into place. A "bolster" or pack is used to prevent these from movement for 5 days, allowing the graft to heal in its new position. Skin grafts are thin and do not have their own blood supply. Instead, tiny blood vessels from the defect grow into the skin graft in the first 5 days which allow the skin graft to survive in its new location. Any movement or fluid collection disrupts this healing process and can cause the graft to die. Skin grafts work very well for many oral cavity tumors and are often used to reconstruct tongue or floor of mouth oral cavity tumors when primary closure would interfere with tongue movement permanently. Skin grafts are also used to line the sinus cavity after sinus surgery for cancer when a prosthesis to reconstruct the teeth is planned. The skin graft can be used to recreate the floor of mouth or allow the remaining tongue to move freely without tethering or restriction. Because our mouths continually make saliva, which can work its way under the skin graft and prevent it from healing in those critical first 5 days, the bolster used to secure the skin graft in oral cavity cancer surgery has to be tied in tightly and may interfere with breathing and eating, depending on the location. Your surgeon may recommend a temporary tracheostomy or feeding tube to protect your airway during this time.

Pedicled flaps

The next most complex form of flap reconstruction is the pedicled flap. This refers to the use of nearby tissue which is inserted into the defect resulting from surgery but remains attached to its own blood supply (the "pedicle"). The flap can consist of muscle alone or muscle plus overlying skin. Some examples of pedicled flaps are the forehead flap, used to reconstruct large nasal defects, or the pectoralis flap, which is a commonly used pedicled flap that uses one of the chest pectoral muscles to reconstruct large defects of the head and neck and can include some overlying skin or just the muscle alone. This is one of the most common flaps used for reconstruction and the flap is tunneled under the skin to the area being reconstructed. Pectoralis flaps can be used to reconstruct oral cavity, oropharynx, larynx, and hypopharynx defects after surgery, as well as being used to reconstruct skin defects of the neck and lower face. In addition, a pectoralis flap can be used to fill in areas of the jaw in patients who require removal of part of the lower jaw (mandible), who are not candidates for free flap reconstruction. These flaps will never function as a jaw replacement, and patients who undergo such reconstruction usually do not have teeth and are restricted to a soft diet, but these flaps can provide a good cosmetic result and coverage. It is important to discuss with your doctor whether or not a metal plate will be used in such circumstances. The failure rate of metal plates is very high, particularly if radiation is used post-operatively and a good result can be accomplished with the use of the pectoralis flap alone for jaw reconstruction.

Free flaps

Free flaps are relatively new in medicine, having only come into wide spread use in the past 20 years. Free flaps entail removing tissue from another part of the body, freeing the tissue completely, and placing it in the head and neck defect. Hence the flaps are "free," without any pedicle. Free flap tissue includes one artery and one or two veins that are attached to the flap. In order for these to survive in their new location, the artery and veins need to be sewn into existing arteries and veins in the head and neck so the flap will have a blood supply. This very fact makes free flaps more complicated than the previous types of reconstruction. Sewing these vessels requires special skill and a microvascular surgeon (a surgeon with specific training in the use of free flaps) and requires a microscope in order to perform this delicate blood vessel repair. A microvascular surgeon is a head and neck surgeon or plastic surgeon who has done specific training in free flap reconstruction. It is important to ask your reconstructive surgeon how many head and neck free flap reconstructions he or she has done because the head and neck is a special area of small spaces. A free flap that is too bulky could permanently interfere with speech, swallowing, and breathing, unlike other areas of the body where the extra tissue may not be a big deal. Free flaps also add significant time to the length of the operation with an average of at least 6 additional hours in most cases. Patients with other medical problems, such as heart trouble, may not be candidates for a free flap reconstruction because the additional time under anesthesia can worsen those other problems and make that length of surgery dangerous. In addition, patients with poor circulation may not be candidates for a free flap because the free flap includes removing not only tissue but an artery and one to two veins. If the artery is the one that provides most of the blood flow to your leg or arm, removing it for the free flap can result in the loss of a limb.

Patients who undergo free flap reconstruction can expect to spend approximately 2 to 3 days in intensive care afterwards. This is because you will need more close monitoring in the initial post-operative period after having had such a long surgery and also because the free flap will require close monitoring (hourly checks) by your treatment team during these first few days to make sure the sutured vessels do not form a clot or go into spasm. If this happens, your surgeon will take you back to the operating room to explore the vessels and remove any clot. You will be placed on dextran and heparin post-operatively to thin your blood and minimize the chance of clotting. The actual length of stay for all reconstructive procedures varies greatly depending on where the tumor is located and the type of reconstruction performed and should be discussed with your doctor beforehand.

The most commonly used free flaps for head and neck reconstruction are the radial forearm free flap, the lateral thigh free flap, and the fibula free flap. Other flaps that can be used include the lateral arm free flap (a skin and soft tissue flap from the side of the upper arm, above the elbow), the latissimus dorsi free flap (a muscle from the side), the rectus abdominus free flap (the rectus muscle from the wall of the abdomen, with or without overlying skin), the iliac crest free flap (bone with or without muscle from the hip) and the scapula free flap (a muscle and bone flap from the back of the shoulder). Jejunal free flaps use a segment of small intestine for reconstruction of the pharynx and upper esophagus for advanced larynx and hypopharynx tumors to recreate a swallowing tube. These require an intra-abdominal incision and are associated with a longer recovery period as a result.

Radial forearm free flap

This flap comes from the undersurface of the lower arm, below the elbow. If you pinch your skin there, you will find that it is thin and soft. This makes it a good flap for complex oral cavity defects, oropharyngeal defects, and increasingly these are being used in laryngectomy surgery if there is not enough tissue to close primarily without interfering with swallowing or if you have had prior radiation. A segment of the radius bone and some muscle can also be removed with the radius flap to allow bony reconstruction of small bone defects, such as the upper jaw (maxilla). The arm defect is covered with a skin graft to protect the muscles and tendons. Make sure your surgeon is aware if you are right-handed or left-handed as he or she will use the non-dominant arm for the radial artery free flap. Because there is a risk of nerve or tendon injury, patients who depend on their hands for a living, such as musicians, may not be good candidates for a radial forearm free flap.

Fibular free flap

The fibular free flap is primarily used for reconstruction of the mandible or lower jaw. The fibula is a long, thin bone in the lower leg below the knee that can be removed with usually no long-term effects on weight bearing, because the larger tibia bone in the lower leg is left undisturbed. Overlying muscle and skin can be removed intact with the fibula to provide surface coverage of complex oral cavity defects. The peroneal artery is the artery that is removed, or harvested, with the fibular free flap to provide a blood supply to the flap after it is anastomosed or sutured to blood vessels in the neck. Patients who are being considered for fibular free flaps have to have adequate blood flow to the lower leg and foot through other blood vessels, to avoid loss of the leg with removal of the peroneal artery which can happen if that vessel is supplying most of the blood flow to the leg. Therefore patients who have poor circulation may not be candidates for a fibular free flap. As with the radial forearm free flap, there is a risk of nerve and/or tendon injury in the lower leg which can cause problems lifting the foot. Physical therapy is particularly important during the recovery period after fibular free flap reconstruction. Patients are usually placed in a leg boot during the healing process and weight bearing is limited for the first several weeks following surgery. Sometimes the leg wound can be closed primarily, but if muscle and skin are removed along with the fibula, the leg defect is covered with a skin graft to protect the muscles and tendons.

Lateral thigh free flap

The lateral thigh free flap (also called anterolateral thigh free flap) is increasingly gaining in popularity among re-constructive surgeons for head and neck reconstruction. This flap includes skin and soft tissue of the outer part of the upper leg; thigh muscle can be included as well when a thicker flap is required. The advantage of the lateral thigh free flap is that the blood supply is usually reliable and does not have the same risk of nerve or tendon injury that the radius or fibular flaps do. Most of the time, the leg wound can be closed primarily. If the amount of skin and soft tissue removed is large, a skin graft is required to cover the leg wound or "donor site."

PROSTHESIS

In some circumstances, a prosthesis can be an excellent al-ternative to tissue reconstruction and often can give a bet-ter result than a tissue reconstruction. Examples of such cases would be reconstruction of the ear, nose, or eye when these have to be removed to treat cancer. Despite surgical advances, these are areas where surgical reconstruction will never look as real as a prosthesis could (see **Figure 3-1**). These prostheses are made out of silicone or plastic and are held in place by clips, magnets, or adhesive glue. Another area where a prosthesis is an excellent alternative to soft tissue reconstruction is in reconstruction of maxillectomy defects, when part of the upper jaw has to be removed, or to treat soft palate defects. The prosthesis in this case is a modified dental obturator (like a denture) that can include teeth and allows normal speech and swallowing. Unlike a flap, the prosthesis can be easily removed during examinations to monitor for tumor recurrence. The specialists who create facial prosthesis are called anaplastologists, while those who specialize in oral prostheses usually have a dental background in prosthodontics. These specialists are often affiliated with major medical centers and are more commonly found in major cities.

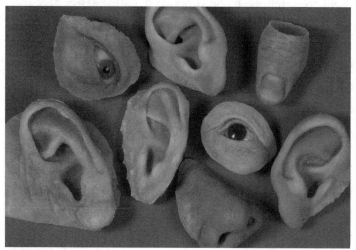

FIGURE 3-1.   Example of prosthetic devices for complex facial defects

Those who desire immediate reconstruction, but for medical reasons are not good candidates for the procedure, need to find peace within themselves about this situation. Talking with other survivors who have experienced the same situation can be very enlightening and useful. Your health care team can connect you with a local support group as well. In some cases, reconstruction can be revisited at the end of treatment and may give you a silver lining to look forward to later. Until then, consider yourself a "work in progress."

RECOVERING FROM SURGERY

Recovery from surgery is easier if you understand what kind of procedure your surgeon will be doing beforehand. Ask your doctor about the details of the specific procedure you will undergo, including the type of incision, exactly what will be removed, and what you will and will not be allowed to do immediately after surgery. This knowledge will help you manage your expectations, care, and recovery.

You will not be allowed to drive for at least 2 weeks after surgery. Arrange to have a family member or friend take you to and from the hospital. In addition, you will need to arrange for someone to stay with you for at least the first 48 hours after surgery. Make sure you have made arrangements to have help at home after surgery for at least 1 week. Expect to need help for several weeks after surgery. The extent of help and the length of time you will need help will vary depending on the extent of your surgery. You may need some assistance at home managing drains for a few days, attending to wound care and such, and recovering from surgery in general. Ask your surgeon what to expect, and request to meet with a nurse to review teaching instructions prior to your surgery date so you are well prepared as to what to expect.

If other people will be coming to stay to help you, talk about roles and responsibilities beforehand. Write out what each person is responsible for doing—buying the groceries, changing bandages, making dinner, taking the kids to soccer practice, and so on. Planning ahead prevents problems later. Accept help during this time. If you over exert yourself, you could negatively impact the wound healing process. Talk with your home caregivers, whether family or friends, about your expectations of each other before surgery. One issue that many families encounter is deciding when the patient should actually look at the incision. The patient needs to be in charge of that decision. Some people are comfortable right away; others delay for some time. Don't delay too long though. It is advisable to talk about this decision in advance and agree on a plan. Gathering information from your surgeon and cancer survivors or looking at photographs in the doctor's office can help to know what to expect.

If your surgery involves drains and wound management at home, decide in advance who will be responsible for helping with emptying the drains and providing the dressing changes. If your family is not comfortable with these tasks or not able to take care of these tasks, your doctor can arrange home health nurse visits. You should receive detailed instructions from your doctor, nurses, and physical therapists about what kind of activity is allowed during the healing period. Make sure you know what you should not be doing! It will be important to get plenty of rest during the recovery process to allow your body to heal and to take pain medication as prescribed by your surgeon. Pain medications can slow down bowel function, so be sure to take stool softeners prescribed by your surgeon for this purpose if you are on an oral diet. It is equally important to move around as much as possible to avoid getting blood clots or pneumonia. Too much time in bed or in one position is a risk factor for both of these complications.

If you have to be fed through a feeding tube during the recovery period, make sure all caregivers are comfortable managing these tubes at home. The idea of a feeding tube scares many people, but actually a feeding tube is just a way of pouring liquid calories directly into your stomach, bypassing your mouth and throat, to allow those areas to heal. Make sure you are comfortable with flushing the feeding tube with water to prevent it from clogging from the high nutrient tube feedings. Your doctor should have a nutritionist meet with you before discharge to review the type of tube feeding prescribed. Some formulas like Ensure or Boost Plus can be obtained from stores, while other types require a prescription. Make sure you know how to take your medications through the feeding tube. Some can be crushed in water, but others may need to be changed. Similarly, tracheostomy care will be taught to you and your caregivers before discharge from the hospital. Make sure you are comfortable with this and are given a portable suction unit for home use before discharge. These post-operative issues are discussed in greater detail in Chapter 4.

Finally, report any unusual symptoms immediately. You will be given a detailed instruction sheet at discharge about what these unusual symptoms may include. However, you know your body better than anyone. If you feel unwell or something doesn't seem right, call your doctor right away.

THE UNASKED QUESTION: RESUMING PHYSICAL INTIMACY AFTER SURGERY

After discharge from the hospital, your doctor or physical therapist will instruct you to do a specific set of exercises to begin regaining arm strength, range of motion, and general physical well-being. However, both physicians and patients tend to overlook one question that is hardly ever asked: When is it safe to resume sexual activity? The timing of when you can resume sexual activities will vary greatly depending on the type of surgery you have. The time frame is usually quite short for patients who do not require reconstruction. With reconstructive surgery, however, you should ask your reconstructive surgeon about which physical activities, including sex, can be resumed and when. Make sure to ask this often unasked question. Sex is a normal and healthy activity. Do not be embarrassed to ask.

You may suffer from feelings of loss of self image, despair, and depression that make you feel unattractive and no longer like a sexual being. You are not alone. It is the rare patient who does not experience some degree of loss after any surgery of the head and neck, even the smallest scar, because it is such an important part of our appearance and how we present ourselves to others. Make sure you communicate these feelings to your partner and your surgeon. To some degree, such feelings are normal and improve as you heal. Talking to members of a head and neck cancer support group may be one of the best forums for sharing such deeply personal feelings, as you are not alone, and fellow survivors understand from personal experience much of what you suffer. However, sometimes these emotions can worsen over time and cause a snowball effect, growing larger and larger. This is not healthy and will interfere with your recovery and cancer battle by draining you of valuable energy you need to fight. There are resources available for you. Some patients benefit from counseling or meeting with a therapist. Depressive symptoms, if persistent, can impact your recovery negatively as well as your quality of life and outlook. Depressive symptoms can be treated so talk to your doctor if they persist.

ADJUVANT TREATMENT AFTER SURGERY

The need for additional treatment in the form of radiation therapy or chemoradiation will depend on the stage of the disease, type of surgery performed, the grade of the cancer cells, the age of the patient, the general health of the patient, and other prognostic factors determined by the pathologist after examining the tumor obtained from surgery. It is routine and should be expected that patients undergoing surgery for most advanced stage head and neck tumors (stage 3 and stage 4) will need radiation therapy post-operatively to help ensure that the cancer doesn't return. In addition, your surgeon may recommend radiation therapy if cancer is found to spread along nerves in the surgical specimen, as this is associated with a higher risk of the tumor coming back, as well as if cancer is found in the cervical (neck) lymph nodes on the pathology report. Some surgeons advise radiation therapy for any positive node, while others recommend radiation therapy if more than one lymph node is involved.

Post-operative radiation is required for any lymph node that demonstrates extracapsular spread on pathologic evaluation. If you think of a lymph node as an egg (although normal lymph nodes are the size of a lentil bean), extracapsular spread refers to a tumor that has broken through the capsule, or shell, of the lymph node. The risk of recurrence is much higher in patients with extracapsular spread, hence the need for radiation therapy post-operatively to kill any remaining cells. Extracapsular spread is also associated with a higher risk of spread to distant sites, such as the lungs. Your surgeon may recommend post-operative chemoradiation in this circumstance. The need for chemotherapy is unrelated to the type of surgery done; it is based on the degree of risk of the cancer returning.

When we actually look at the entire treatment experience from beginning to end for patients needing surgery with post-operative radiation, treatment lasts between 4 to 6 months on average—radiation treatments are started no sooner than 3 weeks after surgery, to give your tissue some time to heal, but no later than 6 weeks after surgery in order not to let any microscopic cancer cells gain a foothold. It takes approximately 6 weeks to give the usual post-operative dose of between 50 to 60 Gy. It will take you another 6 to 8 weeks to recover from the effects of radiation. The effects of radiation are ongoing for approximately the same amount of time that you were in radiation treatment.

NON-OPERATIVE TREATMENT

Non-operative therapy for head and neck cancer consists of radiation therapy, chemoradiation, chemotherapy, or targeted biological therapy. As with surgery, early-stage tumors (stage 1 or 2) can be successfully treated with single modality therapy alone. In the case of head and neck cancer, this means radiation. Advanced-stage tumors (stage 3 and 4) require multimodality therapy, or more than one type of treatment. This can consist of radiation plus chemotherapy or radiation plus a targeted biological drug. Chemotherapy alone is not curative. Finally, some patients may have tumors that are inoperable (removing the tumor surgically may not be possible with a reasonable chance of cure). Inoperable does not mean incurable; it means surgically incurable. In such cases, non-operative therapy is indicated.

The advantage to non-operative therapy is the avoidance of surgery, but radiation and chemotherapy have significant side effects and may have long-term implications for you. Be sure you are fully informed about the risks and benefits of all possible forms of treatment before deciding on a treatment course.

RADIATION

Radiation therapy can be used as primary treatment alone for some early-stage head and neck cancers or in combination with chemotherapy for advanced-stage disease. Many patients with advanced cancer can be successfully treated with non-operative therapy without the need for major surgery. Several well-regarded clinical trials have shown that for stage 3 larynx cancer, chemoradiation is comparable to surgery with post-operative radiation and avoids surgery in two-thirds of patients. This advance is very important, however, physicians and patients alike must resist the temptation to generalize decision making regarding therapy to all patients. For example, in oral cancer, surgery is superior to non-operative therapy. And chemoradiation is never indicated for stage 1 or stage 2 disease simply because it is not required. The side effects are too great, and there are no data to show that adding chemotherapy provides a benefit in early-stage disease.

Radiation therapy uses ionizing radiation to kill cancer cells. X-rays are a type of ionizing radiation, as are gamma rays or protons, however, the doses used to treat cancer are much greater than those used to take an X-ray. Radiation reacts with water molecules in growing cells to form free radicals, which damage the cell's genetic material, or DNA. The faster a cell is growing or dividing, the greater the effect of radiation on the cell. Because cancer cells grow so much more quickly than normal tissue, and can't repair the cellular damage caused by radiation like normal cells can, they are more susceptible to the effects of radiation and treatment, which eventually results in cell death. Radiation does not kill cancer cells right away; it can take weeks before cancer cells start to die. In addition, the effect of radiation is ongoing for a period of time after treatment and cancer cells will continue to die for weeks to months after the end of treatment. Some normal tissues will be affected as well, but because these are normal cells with normal cell repair mechanisms, they can usually recover from the effects of radiation. Scarring of normal tissue with decreased blood flow may occur as a side effect. Cells that are not growing, or cells that grow very slowly, are less affected by radiation. Certain tissues are at greater risk for permanent injury from radiation, such as hair, skin, salivary gland tissue, the jawbone, and the thyroid gland. These are mentioned in greater detail in the section on side effects.

Radiation treatments are in themselves painless and are very much like having an X-ray done. Typically, patients undergoing radiation will first undergo a simulation, where the radiation oncologist will map out the areas to be treated based on your cancer. This simulation is done to ensure that the radiation beams are always lined up the exact same way to radiate the same area consistently and precisely. A few tiny tattoo marks (little blue dots) will be made on your neck as part of the preparation process. These dots are usually permanent. Do not have these dots lasered off later. They are important markings for the future in the event recurrence were to happen or other medical issues arose related to your radiation. A mask is usually made of your face and neck that you will be asked to wear during each treatment, to ensure that your head is in the same position every time you have a radiation treatment so that the treatment targets the planned areas exactly. The mask is made of a plastic mesh that you can breathe through and is well-tolerated.

Treatment is usually delivered through an external beam radiation machine, and the process is very similar to having an X-ray done. The treatments last about 5 minutes and in order to minimize the effects of radiation on normal tissue, the total dose of radiation is divided into fractions, spread out over a 6- to 8-week period. The average dose for radiation given as a curative treatment modality is between 70 and 80 Gy, which is a higher dose than the dose used following surgery. Treatments are given Monday through Friday in either once-daily fractions or twice-daily fractions. Although it means you must go every day to the radiation facility, you are in and out quickly, usually in less than 30 minutes. There have been vast improvements in radiation therapy over the last decade or so. Special technology is used so that only tissues that need to be radiated are exposed to radiation. Ask your radiation oncologist if your tumor can be treated with intensity-modulated radiation therapy (IMRT) or conformal radiation therapy, which are both methods of delivering more highly targeted radiation to the tumor while trying to spare normal surrounding tissue. Both involve conventional radiation, and are best done at centers with a large experience in these techniques. Whether or not you can receive IMRT or conformal radiation depends on where your tumor is, how large it is, and what the risk for local spread is. The side effects are the same as for conventional external beam radiation but may be less intense.

Radiation treatments themselves do not hurt. It feels similar to getting a chest X-ray, which means you feel nothing at all. However radiation has side effects which are cumulative; you may start getting fatigued toward the last few weeks of treatment. Exercising regularly, such as power walking, has proven to reduce this specific side effect.

The areas of your head and neck treated with radiation may become pink or puffy; sometimes the skin may look burned. A sore mouth and sore throat are common during treatment but usually don't occur until halfway through treatment. Many patients start to feel quite discouraged in the third and fourth week of treatment because the side effects start to manifest themselves. It is very important to not give up—consider this a sign that the radiation is working. It is also important to try to swallow every day if your physician or swallowing therapist says this is safe, even if your throat is sore and you don't feel like it. The muscles used in swallowing, like any other muscle, need to be used or they are prone to scarring from the radiation.

For some people, the effects of radiation can last quite some time, with the tissue of the neck and throat going through subtle changes for as along as a year after treatment is completed. Your skin and tissues may feel firmer and be tanner looking or puffy for an extended period of time or even shrink a little and feel stiff. Swallowing troubles can increase as time passes, because of gradual stiffening of the muscles of the throat and pharynx. Swallowing therapy is helpful in treating and preventing this problem.

SIDE EFFECTS

Knowing what to expect can help you to deal with the expected side effects of radiation therapy. Radiation has some specific side effects that occur commonly. Hair, skin, and salivary gland tissue are commonly affected by radiation because these tend to be faster growing tissues. It is common for men to lose their beard in areas of the neck or face that receive radiation, and this hair usually does not grow back. Your skin can get dry and burned from radiation treatments. The skin usually recovers, and your radiation oncologist will advise you on how to treat and protect your skin. Over the counter skin cleansers and lotions for sensitive skin, such as Cetaphil®, are good choices to replace soap and perfume-based lotions. It is good to avoid direct sun exposure of those areas that receive radiation to avoid permanent darkening; if you must be outdoors, use a zinc-oxide-based sunscreen. Finally, the normal cells that line the mouth and the salivary glands are affected by radiation. Mucositis, or inflammation of the lining of the mouth and throat, commonly occurs during radiation. Your mouth may feel raw, and spicy or acidic foods (like oranges or tomatoes) or firm crunchy foods will make it feel worse. Your mouth will recover. Your doctor will prescribe oral rinses to soothe your mouth; avoiding irritating foods helps manage symptoms.

Dry mouth

Salivary gland tissue, which has a fast growth rate, is permanently affected by doses of radiation used to cure cancer. This can result in dry mouth, also called xerostomia, and this is unfortunately permanent. Xerostomia requires lifelong supportive treatment with over-the-counter dry mouth topical artificial saliva preparations (Biotene® and MouthKote® are examples). Most patients find they have to carry a water bottle with them at all times to replace the moisture their mouth no longer makes. In some cases, radiation can be targeted to protect some of the salivary gland tissue in an effort to avoid this permanent side effect. Salivary gland transfer is an experimental procedure being studied to see if at least one salivary gland can be moved (transferred) out of the area to be radiated. This is not appropriate for all patients and you need to make sure you aren't at risk for cancer in the areas containing the salivary glands before consenting to this procedure.

Swallowing difficulty

Your doctor may recommend a feeding tube before undergoing radiation treatment. For most patients, this is temporary, and the feeding tube can be removed after treatment is completed. Some people have swallowing trouble because of the cancer and are unable to take adequate nutrition. Because radiation can cause a sore throat or make existing swallowing problems worse, a feeding tube is an important adjunct to your treatment during this critical time. If you are unable to take in adequate calories and liquids during treatment because you are unable to swallow, you can get dehydrated and radiation treatments may need to be interrupted to give your body a chance to recover. These interruptions in treatment are called "treatment breaks" and are best avoided because when you give your body a break, you are also giving the cancer a break and a chance to recover. Feeding tubes can be inserted through into your stomach or directly through the stomach percutaneous gastrostomy tube or PEG tube. A PEG requires a small surgical procedure to place, but many patients find this more comfortable. A PEG avoids the irritation of the tissues of the nose and throat that a feeding tube placed through the nose can cause, which can be particularly irritating if those tissues are being exposed to radiation. The average weight loss during head and neck radiation treatments is 30 pounds. If you cannot afford to lose 30 pounds, a feeding tube is valuable, because you can supplement the foods you take in by mouth with tube feedings given through the feeding tube.

Having a feeding tube does not mean you cannot eat. In fact, for most patients, it is important to go on eating if your physician or swallowing therapist says this is safe, even if your throat is sore and you don't feel like it. The muscles used in swallowing, like any other muscle, need to be used or they may develop scarring from the radiation. The importance of working with a speech language pathologist, also known as a swallowing therapist, before, during, and after radiation therapy for head and neck cancer cannot be overstated. There is scientific data that shows that patients who work with a swallowing therapist throughout their cancer treatment and afterward, have better swallowing function and quality of life. The swallowing therapist is an important part of your treatment team. Ideally you will be introduced to him or her before you start treatment and will work with them during and after treatment. Because the effects of radiation are ongoing for several months after your last radiation treatment, your swallowing therapy will not end with the end of radiation. In fact, most swallowing difficulties due to radiation occur months after radiation treatment, so it will be important to have scheduled treatment sessions with your swallowing therapist long after your cancer treatment is completed.

Dental issues

One specific effect of head and neck radiation that needs special mention is the effect of radiation on your teeth and jaws. Radiation therapy has permanent effects on the blood supply to the jawbones, as well as to the salivary gland tissue. Saliva contains enzymes that help protect against cavity formation. When you make less saliva, the risk of cavities rises significantly, and so you need to take extra care of your teeth for life following radiation. It is very important to have a thorough dental evaluation prior to beginning radiation treatments to the head and neck. Your dentist will look for any tooth problems, and these should be corrected prior to radiation (as soon as possible). If you have teeth that are in bad condition, these either need to be repaired or extracted before you start radiation because if you require dental surgery after radiation, there is a risk of the jawbone surrounding the teeth not healing properly because the radiation impairs the blood supply to the bone. Dental surgery performed on radiated bone can result in chronic infection and is a devastating complication called osteoradionecrosis, which can result in necrosis or death of all or part of the mandible. In severe cases, removal of the jawbone is required. Therefore any dental work should be completed before you start radiation.

Ask your dentist to make fluoride trays for you. He or she will take an impression of your teeth and make a tray that you place fluoride gel in and wear once or twice a day, for 10 minutes. This needs to become a lifelong habit to help prevent cavities from forming because, again, the loss of saliva from radiation can lead to cavity development. If you need to have your teeth extracted before treatment, have this done as soon as possible because your radiation oncologist will have to delay the start of radiation for 2 to 3 weeks to give your gums a chance to heal. You should increase the frequency of dentist visits to every 3 months for a cleaning instead of once or twice a year. Finally, if you require dental work after radiation, make sure your dentist or oral surgeon is in close contact with your head and neck surgeon. Pre-treatment with hyperbaric oxygen (a treatment where you are exposed to high atmospheric oxygen pressures in a special tank) that is continued post-operatively, as well as long-term antibiotic therapy starting before treatment with oral antibiotics that are effective against normal mouth bacteria and penetrate bone such as clindamycin, are important aids in trying to prevent the devastating complication of osteoradionecrosis. The hyperbaric oxygen treatments force additional oxygen into the radiated bone, which helps the bone to heal from dental surgery. Radiated bone has a lower oxygen content than normal, which allows normal bacteria to set up an infection once the bone is cut into, which happens with dental surgery; infection can be hard to control because of the poor blood supply to radiated bone.

Some people choose to pursue dental implants for tooth restoration after treatment. Because the implants are surgically implanted into the bone, this procedure carries the same risk of osteoradionecrosis that any other dental surgery does after radiation. Make sure your providers communicate with each other before you undergo any elective or emergent dental surgery. Complications of osteoradionecrosis are managed by head and neck surgeons, therefore even if you undergo non-operative treatment for cancer, your surgeon remains an important part of your treatment team and should be consulted before any dental surgery.

Hypothyroidism

Radiation therapy may also damage your thyroid gland. Approximately 60% of people who undergo radiation therapy to the head and neck experience hypothyroidism, or low thyroid hormone levels, as a result of radiation injury to the thyroid gland. Symptoms of hypothyroidism include weight gain, fatigue or lack of energy, depression, constipation, feeling cold, dry or brittle hair, hair loss, dry skin, and hoarseness. These symptoms usually don't occur until after the end of radiation and may take months to develop. Your doctor should monitor you for hypothyroidism, which can easily be detected with simple blood tests.

Smoking

The side effects of radiation are made worse by cigarette smoking, and there is a significant amount of scientific data that shows that patients who smoke during radiation treatment have more severe side effects. In addition, their tumors don't respond as well to treatment with radiation therapy. This effect is directly smoking-related: this effect occurs while you smoke, not because you used to smoke. Please talk to your doctor about smoking cessation help. This is an ideal time to quit for so many reasons, but perhaps the most important is that smoking will interfere with treatment as you battle your head and neck cancer.

CHEMOTHERAPY

The addition of chemotherapy to radiation treatment, called chemoradiation, has been increasingly used since initial clinical trials in the 1990s showed that chemoradiation was comparable to surgery with post-operative radiation for patients with stage 3 advanced laryngeal cancer. Such patients formerly were only offered surgery with post-operative radiation; radiation alone was less effective than when combined with surgery to treat advanced head and neck cancer. The findings of these studies, and numerous large institutional studies performed since then, have ushered in a new era for patients with head and neck cancer, many of whom can be treated with organ-preserving non-operative therapy with chemoradiation.

Chemotherapy refers to drugs that are cytotoxic—that is, they cause cell death. There are many different types of chemotherapy drugs, all with different mechanisms of action that result in tumor cell death. The most commonly used drugs to treat head and neck cancer are cisplatin, carboplatin, 5-fluorouracil (5-FU), and taxol. These can be given alone or in combination. Chemotherapy drugs alone are not curative in the treatment of head and neck cancer. Though these drugs can result in impressive initial tumor shrinkage, the drugs may not reach cells in the middle of the tumor mass. In addition, tumor cells vary in their response to chemotherapy. The less "normal" a cancer cell is, the less likely it is that the cells use normal cell growth patterns to divide and grow, and therefore the drug may not be effective. Head and neck cancers are clever and can change and become resistant to chemotherapy when given over time so that eventually the tumor will recur.

Chemotherapy has been shown to increase the effect of radiation on tumor cells when used with radiation therapy. Chemotherapy acts as a radiosensitizer, making cancer cells more sensitive to the effects of radiation. It is indicated for patients with advanced-stage head and neck cancers who are at high risk for recurrance and distant metastases. Initial studies used a type of chemoradiation called induction chemotherapy, where three courses of chemotherapy were administered several weeks apart, and those patients who had a response then went on to receive radiation, while those cancers that didn't respond were treated with surgery and radiation. Some medical oncologists still use induction chemotherapy regimens, but more commonly chemotherapy is given concurrently with radiation therapy, either as weekly treatments or for a total of three treatments during the 6- to 8-week course of radiation therapy. This is called concurrent or concomitant chemoradiation and is based on studies showing improved tumor response rates with this approach.

The radiosensitizing effect of chemotherapy on radiation means that the side effects of chemoradiation are greater than for radiation alone. All of the side effects associated with radiation can occur; however, the mucositis of the tissues lining the mouth and throat is more severe, and swallowing difficulties both during and after treatment may be more severe in intensity and duration. Chemotherapy also has its own set of side effects depending on the drug used, including hair loss, gastrointestinal symptoms, and fatigue. Not all chemotherapy drugs cause hair loss. Talk with your medical oncologist about what steps can be taken to reduce possible side effects from chemotherapy. Not everyone experiences side effects today. Medications are available to prevent or dramatically reduce nausea. Exercise has been proven to help reduce the side effect of fatigue. During your chemotherapy, your blood will be taken at designated intervals to make sure that your red blood cells and white blood cells are staying within normal limits. If they are low, which is a common side effect, the doctor might decide to give you special medicines to boost your blood counts back up to a normal range. Be careful to avoid being around people who have a cold or flu as your immune system is being taxed during treatment.

Because chemoradiation carries a one-two punch, the mucositis and sore throat may be worse than with radiation alone, and nausea from some chemotherapy drugs can limit oral intake. Many patients undergoing chemoradiation will need a feeding tube or PEG placed before treatment as a preventive measure. Think of it as an insurance policy. Again, you don't have to use it and it is preferable to swallow by mouth whenever possible, but it is there if you need it. It is important to address the issue of the feeding tube or PEG before starting chemotherapy. Because chemotherapy drugs can lower your white blood cell count, it is unwise to have a PEG placed within 1 month of a chemotherapy treatment. If you get an infection at the site or have a complication, your body will not be able to fight back normally to heal. In such cases, a feeding tube through the nose, while uncomfortable, is safer.

Chemotherapy is administered through intravenous infusion in an oncology clinic while you relax in a chair. You will be monitored for side effects for several hours afterwards. Your oncologist may recommend that you have an infusaport placed, which is an indwelling intravenous catheter placed in a large vein. This is helpful if the chemotherapy drugs used are irritating to smaller veins, if you are going to receive weekly chemotherapy treatments, or you have difficulties with intravenous catheter placement. Only the infusaport has to be stuck in the future, not you, and it can be removed after your treatment is completed.

Most patients feel well the day of the treatment. If side effects occur, they most commonly happen the night of chemotherapy or the next day. Focus on what chemotherapy is designed to do FOR you—destroy any cancer cells that have spread elsewhere in the body. Use visual imagery to picture how these drugs work and focus on those images while actually receiving the drugs. Celebrate the completion of each cycle of treatment. Remember you are climbing further up the survival cure by taking chemotherapy. Take pride in this victory. It's important to realize that some patients may react differently to chemotherapy than others do. Talking with other head and neck cancer survivors who have had the same chemotherapy drugs will not really answer the question for you in advance of how you personally are going to feel and what side effects you may or may not experience. Remember, too, that there is a beginning and an end to taking chemotherapy. We can deal with anything when we know it is for a designated period of time. When something has no known end in sight is when it gets much harder to cope with.

Chemoradiation is not appropriate for patients who have early-stage cancer. In these cases, when the risk of metastatic disease is low, there is no evidence to support a benefit from chemotherapy, and it is more dangerous to over-treat patients. Age is also a factor in deciding who is appropriate to receive chemotherapy and who may not benefit. Elderly, frail patients, for example, may be advised that chemotherapy would not be wise for them to embark on because the side effects of chemotherapy may just be too risky to their life.

You may ask if there are special circumstances in which chemotherapy is actually recommended as the first phase of treatment against head and neck cancer. There is no evidence to support giving chemotherapy alone for definitive treatment of head and neck cancer, unlike other types of cancer. Because chemotherapy in head and neck cancer is used as an adjunct to curative treatment and is not itself curative, there is no evidence that delaying surgery or radiation in order to give chemotherapy first increases the likelihood of the patient being able to have less surgery or radiation than originally anticipated. No benefit has been shown, and the risks of delaying definitive treatment are too high.

Chemotherapy may be used as the only treatment in patients who develop recurrence or metastases after failure of other treatment such as surgery or radiation. In such cases, treatment is not intended to be curative, but to treat symptoms and control tumor growth. This approach, called palliative chemotherapy, is discussed in greater detail in Chapter 9.

TARGETED BIOLOGICAL THERAPY

Erbitux is a monoclonal antibody that binds to the epidermal growth factor receptor (EGFR), which is present on the surface of some cells, and plays a role in regulating cell growth. Epidermal growth factors normally bind to the EGFR receptor to stimulate cells to grow. By binding to the EGFR receptor, Erbitux interferes with the growth of cancer cells by preventing normal growth factors from binding to cancer cells and stimulating cell growth. This targeted biological therapy is not the same thing as conventional chemotherapy, which is meant to kill cells. Erbitux is not directly cytotoxic (causing cell death) but instead indirectly causes cell death by preventing cells from growing and reproducing.

Antibodies are substances that are produced by the immune system in response to a foreign substance such as a bacteria, virus, or toxin. They are the body's natural defense mechanism against infection and help to destroy infectious agents. Monoclonal antibodies are antibodies produced in a laboratory to target a very specific portion of foreign substances. Because they are so specific, ideally treatment with such targeted biological therapy has fewer side effects. Erbitux is given intravenously and can cause serious side effects, which may include difficulty in breathing, low blood pressure, and stiffening of the lungs (interstitial lung disease). Less serious but common side effects include a skin rash (acne, rash, dry skin), fatigue (tiredness, weakness), fever, constipation, and abdominal pain. Skin rash is commonly seen and may predict a better response to treatment with Erbitux. Think of the rash as proof that the drug is working.

Erbitux is a relatively new drug which was first developed for the treatment of colon cancer. To date, studies comparing Erbitux have compared it to radiation therapy alone, rather than chemoradiation. There appears to be a survival advantage when Erbitux is combined with radiation, when compared to radiation alone for patients with advanced-stage tumors. It has not been compared to standard chemoradiation, which is known to be superior to radiation alone for advanced disease. To date, the use of Erbitux is usually confined to patients who cannot undergo chemotherapy for medical reasons, because of fewer and less severe side effects. Your medical oncologist will decide if Erbitux is appropriate in your case. Erbitux is the only targeted biological agent available for treatment of head and neck cancer, but other drugs are currently being tested in clinical trials and hopefully will be available for use one day.

CLINICAL TRIALS

New and innovative treatments are developed and implemented through clinical trials. Without clinical trials we could not improve the treatment of head and neck cancer, nor could we develop ways to prevent it in the future. Clinical trials are the backbone of science today. Anticipate that your doctor will discuss what clinical trials you may be a candidate to consider. Be open-minded. Hear what is being offered as part of a study. Clinical trials are research studies in which people agree to try new therapies under careful supervision in order to help doctors identify the best treatments with the fewest side effects. These studies help improve the overall standard of care for the future. Clinical trials may provide you an edge over standard treatment and in the future may actually become the new method of treatment for people diagnosed with head and neck cancer after you.

There are many different kinds of clinical trials. They range from studies focusing on ways to prevent, detect, diagnosis, treat, and control head and neck cancer, to studies that address quality of life issues that affect our patients. Most clinical trials are carried out in phases. Each phase is designed to learn different information and build upon the information previously discovered. Patients may be eligible for studies in different phases depending on their stage of disease, therapies anticipated, as well as treatment they have already had. Patients are monitored at specific intervals while participating in studies too.

PHASE I STUDIES

Phase I studies are used to find the best way to do a new treatment and how much of it can be given safely. In such studies only a small number of patients are asked to participate. These studies are offered to patients whose cancer cannot be helped by other known treatment modalities. These patients are battling metastatic cancer and have usually exhausted other treatment options. Some patients have personally received benefit from participation but others have experienced no benefit in fighting their cancer. They are, however, paving the way for the next generation by helping physicians to test new drugs, which is important. Once the optimum dose is chosen, the drug is studied for its ability to shrink tumors in phase II trials.

PHASE II STUDIES

Phase II studies are designed to find out if the treatment actually kills cancer cells in patients. A slightly larger cohort of patients is selected for this trial, usually between 20 and 50. Patients whose cancer has no longer responded to other known treatments may be offered participation in this type of trial. Tumor shrinkage is measured and patients are closely observed to measure the effects the treatment is having on treating the disease. If at least 20% of patients in this study respond to treatment, the treatment is considered to be successful. Side effects are also closely monitored and carefully recorded and addressed.

PHASE III STUDIES

Phase III studies usually compare standard treatments already in use with treatments that appeared to be good in small cohort phase II trials. This level requires large numbers, usually thousands, of patients to participate. Patients are usually randomized for the treatment regimen they will be receiving. These studies are seeking benefits of longer survival, better quality of life, fewer side effects, and few cases of cancer recurrence. This is the most common type of clinical trial you may hear about and be offered to participate in.

ADJUVANT STUDIES

Adjuvant studies are conducted to determine if additional therapy will further improve the chance for long-term survival and reduction in risk of recurrence. This study progresses through phase I, II, and III trials like other treatment studies.

SUPPORTIVE CARE STUDIES

Supportive care studies are tailored to improve ways of managing side effects caused by treatment. They also include some quality of life studies as well.

PREVENTION STUDIES

Prevention studies focus on patients at high risk for developing head and neck cancer or those at risk for a recurrence of disease. These studies commonly are geared toward one group in the cohort taking a medication or some type of therapy and the other arm of the study not receiving anything or receiving a placebo. There are also some studies that focus on early detection and methods of diagnosing cancer sooner when cells begin the process of transforming into a cancer cell before it becomes actual cancer.

Below is a list of questions that you should consider asking your physician. The answers you get may help guide you while decision making and fact finding about clinical trials associated with high-risk status or head and neck cancer diagnosis and treatment:

- What is the purpose of the study?

- How many people will be included in the study?

- What does the study involve? What kind of tests and treatment will I have?

- How are treatments given and what side effects might I expect?

- What are the risks and benefits of each protocol?

- How long will the study last?

- What type of long-term follow-up care is provided for those who participate?

- Will I incur any costs? Will my insurance company pay for part of this?

- When will the results be known?

A patient may derive substantial benefit from participating in clinical trials. Every successful cancer treatment being used today started as a clinical trial. Those patients who participated in these studies were the first to benefit.

Participation can therefore potentially benefit you, and perhaps equally important (and to some more important), may contribute in a major way for the next generation having to deal with this disease.

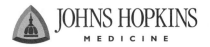

CHAPTER 4

BE PREPARED—THE SIDE
EFFECTS OF TREATMENT

Carol S. Maragos, MSN, CRNP, CNOR
Heather M. Starmer, MA, MS, CCC-SLP
Kimberly Webster, MA, MS, CCC-SLP
Christine G. Gourin, MD, FACS

H ead and neck cancer treatment varies greatly from patient to patient, depending on the primary site and stage of your tumor and whether or not you have previously had treatment. This book will not go into detail about the different types of surgery used to treat cancer of the head and neck; the extent of surgery varies from patient to patient. However, we will cover some of the most common surgical procedures and side effects that you may encounter as part of your treatment. Use these as a starting point for further discussion with your doctor.

Whether your cancer treatment involves surgery, radiation, chemotherapy, or some combination of those three, you may require additional procedures to help with breathing and getting adequate nutrition. Your doctors and ancillary care team will explain the need for these procedures and help you to deal with them along the way. For many of you, the effects of these procedures will be temporary. While it may seem overwhelming at first, you will come to understand the need for these procedures and learn how to manage until they are no longer required. A tracheostomy and a gastrostomy (feeding tube) are two common procedures that many head and neck cancer patients undergo before or during their treatment.

SURGERY

Before undergoing any surgical procedure, we recommend that patients gather all important numbers and contact information and keep it close during your recovery. A sample of such a list of **Important Numbers and Information** is provided at the end of this chapter. In addition, it is important to check your home environment prior to undergoing surgery to make sure you have a safe environment to recover in when you return home. No matter how "minor" the procedure, the effect of anesthesia and pain medications, not to mention surgery, can make you vulnerable to slips and falls. A sample of a **Home Environment Safety Checklist** we recommend is shown at the end of this chapter. Remember that you will not be able to drive for 2 weeks after any major surgery on your neck, and not while you are taking pain medications so it is important to make sure you have all necessary supplies at home before you have surgery as well as contacting people who can help you in case of an emergency in advance.

Prior to surgery, we recommend that patients work through the following list to make sure they are adequately prepared (see **Figure 4-1**). A medic alert tag can be lifesaving to anyone with life- threatening drug allergies or who will have a laryngectomy. Your medic alert tag should be ordered before you undergo the procedure.

If you smoke, now is the time to quit. Your doctor or therapist can provide resources to help you quit. Smoking can interfere with healing, and it has been shown that patients

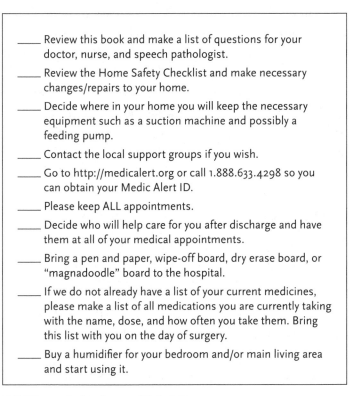

_____ Review this book and make a list of questions for your doctor, nurse, and speech pathologist.

_____ Review the Home Safety Checklist and make necessary changes/repairs to your home.

_____ Decide where in your home you will keep the necessary equipment such as a suction machine and possibly a feeding pump.

_____ Contact the local support groups if you wish.

_____ Go to http://medicalert.org or call 1.888.633.4298 so you can obtain your Medic Alert ID.

_____ Please keep ALL appointments.

_____ Decide who will help care for you after discharge and have them at all of your medical appointments.

_____ Bring a pen and paper, wipe-off board, dry erase board, or "magnadoodle" board to the hospital.

_____ If we do not already have a list of your current medicines, please make a list of all medications you are currently taking with the name, dose, and how often you take them. Bring this list with you on the day of surgery.

_____ Buy a humidifier for your bedroom and/or main living area and start using it.

FIGURE 4-1. Before Surgery: "To Do" List

with head and neck cancer who continue to smoke have an increased risk of tumor recurrence.

Finally, before starting cancer treatment it is important to visit your dentist and make sure any dental issues are addressed. Radiation causes dry mouth (xerostomia), which increases cavity development, and also interferes with the blood supply to the jaws. Therefore, if dental surgery is required, this is best addressed *before* radiation therapy. Ask your dentist for fluoride trays. A fluoride gel can be placed in these trays, which look like tooth guards, and worn once a day to help prevent cavities after radiation. If you find you need dental surgery after you have received radiation therapy, make sure you check with your cancer doctor first before having any procedures done. If the dental work requires some surgery on the jaw bone, you may benefit from hyperbaric oxygen before surgery to prevent infection and loss of the bone, a devastating complication called osteoradionecrosis which can be exacerbated by oral surgery in radiated patients. This side effect and other side effects of radiation are also discussed in Chapter 3.

TRACHEOSTOMY

A tracheostomy is a temporary breathing hole in your neck (see **Figure 4-2**). A tracheostomy tube is inserted to keep your airway open as you recover from surgery.

This tube is placed into your airway in the neck during your surgery and is left in place until the swelling has gone down, usually for several weeks but sometimes longer. You will need to learn how to take care of this breathing tube

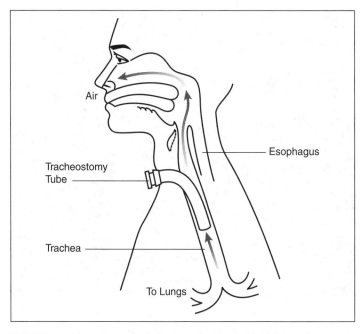

FIGURE 4-2. A tracheostomy tube is a tube inserted into the trachea (windpipe) below the vocal cords to allow unobstructed breathing. *(Figure used with permission of the American Head and Neck Society)*

before you go home (see **Figure 4-3**). The nurses will teach you and a family member or loved one how to suction and clean the tracheostomy tube. Nurses will also help you to order a portable suction machine and supplies for home (see **Figure 4-4**).

WHAT CHANGES SHOULD I EXPECT AFTER A TRACHEOSTOMY?

Breathing

You will be breathing through the tracheostomy tube in your neck, not through the nose and mouth. Breathing will feel different also because your nose and mouth usually

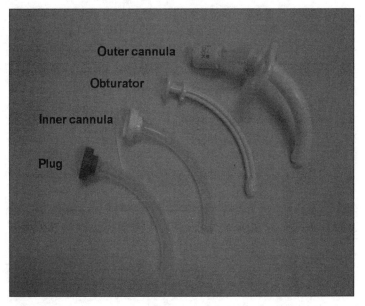

FIGURE 4-3. The tracheostomy tube contains an outer cannula which is placed in the trachea or windpipe, an inner cannula that can be easily removed to remove mucous without removing the whole tube. If the whole tube is removed, the obturator is used to replace the tube. The plug is used to "cap" the tracheostomy tube as a test to see if you can breathe without it prior to removal. You cannot breathe through the tracheostomy tube with a cap on, so this should ONLY be used under your doctor's direction.

warm and moisten your air. When you have a tracheostomy tube your air may be colder and dryer which may irritate your airway. This may lead to coughing or increased mucus production in your windpipe.

Coughing

You will cough through your tracheostomy tube. Some of the mucus may come out of your mouth as well. So be sure to cover your tube and mouth when you cough.

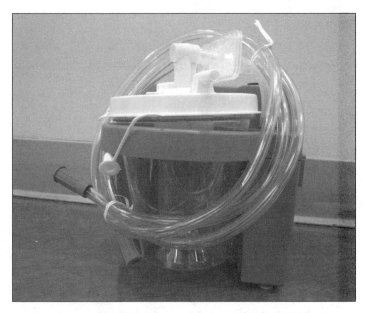

FIGURE 4-4. Every patient with a tracheostomy tube is sent home with a suction device, as shown above, to help with clearing secretions from your airway.

Blowing your nose/sniffing through your nose

Because you will no longer be able to move air through your nose, you will have difficulty blowing your nose and sniffing. There are some techniques you can learn in the future from the speech pathologist to briefly sniff though your nose.

Taste

Food may taste differently after your surgery. This is largely because of the changes in your sense of smell; smell sensation is lost when you are not breathing through your nose.

Eating

Swallowing might be a little slower or more difficult after surgery, but most people return to a normal diet with help from a speech pathologist.

Speaking

Following surgery, you will be unable to speak the way you did before surgery. This is because the tracheostomy tube is placed below the voice box. As a result, air does not pass through the vocal cords. After your operation, you will be able to communicate with a paper and pen or with a communication board. In the early days after surgery, you will use non-oral communication such as pen/paper, Magic Slate, picture board, and pointing. These methods are slower than speaking and can be frustrating to use. Try to be patient during this time. After about 3 to 5 days, the first tracheostomy tube, which contains a cuff or balloon around the outside, will be changed for a tracheostomy tube without a cuff. This will allow you to speak easier. You may also be given a speaking valve called a Passy-Muir valve (see **Figure 4-5**). This valve fits on the end of the tracheostomy tube to allow you to speak "hands-free." If you don't use a Passy-Muir valve, you will need to put your finger at the end of the tracheostomy tube to talk.

Bearing down

It might be more difficult to hold your breath and push down (as for a bowel movement or exercise) after surgery. You may require a stool softener.

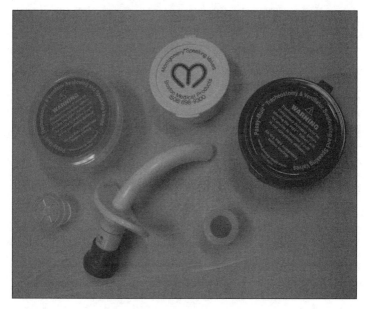

FIGURE 4-5. A Passe-Muir valve. This fits on the end of the trach tube and is a one-way valve that lets air in through the trach tube and closes when you exhale, allowing air to pass out through your vocal cords and mouth. This helps you to talk with a trach tube in.

Your doctor and nurse will provide you with detailed care instructions to take care of your tracheostomy. Additional information can be found on the following web site http://www.hopkinsmedicine.org/tracheostomy/about/index.html. The sections on tracheostomy tube care may be helpful to you regardless of whether or not your tracheostomy tube was placed to treat oral, pharynx, or larynx cancer.

STOMA

If you are having a total laryngectomy, the hole for breathing in your neck will be permanent. It is commonly called a stoma. You may not need a tube in it to keep it open, but it is important to wear a breathable filter over it and to clean it daily. Your nurses and speech pathologist can help you order commercially available stoma covers and filters and teach you how to clean it.

HOW DO I TAKE A SHOWER WITH A TRACHEOSTOMY OR STOMA?

Because your tracheostomy tube or stoma is a direct window to your windpipe and lungs, you will need to be sure water does not enter the hole when bathing. Below are some tips for safe showering. It is important to remember that your stoma/trach should not be fully submerged during bathing or swimming due to potential for drowning.

1. Order a commercially available shower guard. You may be given one in the hospital.

2. Hold a damp washcloth above your stoma.

3. Use a baby bib backwards with the plastic on the outside.

You will be able to wash your hair and all parts of your body as long as the stoma does not get any water into it. See **Figure 4-6** for examples of stoma covers.

HOW DO I CLEAN MY STOMA?

The stoma is to be cleaned often to prevent redness, soreness, and infection of the neck skin. It is also performed to keep the stoma clear of mucus that can make breathing dif-

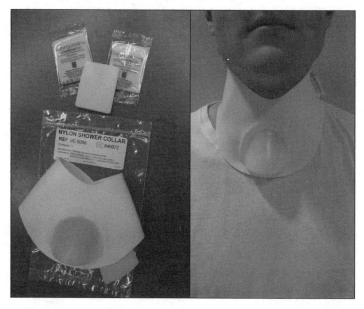

FIGURE 4-6. Examples of stoma covers.

ficult. Clean at least twice a day, more often if you have a lot of mucus, any redness of the skin, or odor from the area.

Supplies

1. Hydrogen peroxide and sterile salt water (50/50 mix)

2. 4×4 gauze

3. Q-tips

4. Tweezers

5. Soap, water, clean washcloths, and tweezers

Instructions

1. Remove the stoma cover.

2. Wash your hands.

3. Look at your skin. Report any increased redness or bleeding to your doctor or nurse.

4. From the time of the surgery until the stoma has healed, you will clean the stoma using sterile gauze or Q-tips and a 50/50 mixture of hydrogen peroxide and sterile salt water (saline). At home, after the stitches are out and the stoma has healed, you may use a clean cloth with soap and water for cleaning the stoma.

5. Start at the hole (stoma) and wipe away from it. Use Q-tips or gauze for one wipe only.

6. Make sure the peroxide solution or soap is rinsed off with water or saline.

7. Use tweezers if needed to pick any dry or crusted mucus from the top of the stoma.

8. Gently pat your skin dry with a dry cloth.

9. Wash the tweezers with warm soap and water after each use. Disinfect them by wiping them off with rubbing alcohol each day.

PEG/FEEDING TUBE

Having proper nutrition is one of the most important parts of recovery and is vitally important to your health during cancer treatment including radiation and chemotherapy. You may have a feeding tube placed during surgery or before starting radiation or chemotherapy. This tube will be used to give you liquid nutrition if you are unable to take enough nutrition by mouth. The tube may be temporary or permanent. The length of time the feeding tube stays in place depends on your healing and length of cancer treatment. You and your family or loved one will be taught how to care for this tube and how to give yourself tube feedings. The tube is often placed in your stomach after a procedure called percutaneous endoscopic gastrostomy or PEG. Occasionally if the tube will only be needed for several days, it may be placed through your nose. This type is called a nasogastric tube or NG tube. Patients and family members are taught how to use and clean the tubes prior to leaving the hospital.

Although you may not feel like eating, proper nutrition is important during cancer treatment. If any food or liquid upsets your stomach or your bowels, let your doctor know. Your weight will be watched very closely. Your dietician and speech pathologist can help you decide the best amounts and types of food and safest way to eat. You may use a combination of eating by mouth and tube feedings.

When you are eating by mouth, it is important for you to report any swallowing trouble, pain with swallowing, new feeling in your throat, or unexplained weight loss to your doctor right away.

NECK DISSECTION

A neck dissection involves removal of the lymph nodes from your neck. This can be a selective removal of lymph nodes when microscopic disease is suspected or comprehensive removal of all of the lymph node tissue in your neck if you have visible lymph node involvement at the time of your cancer diagnosis. Your surgeon may also remove other structures at the time of neck dissection, including the sternocleidomastoid muscle, the internal jugular vein, and the spinal accessory nerve if these are involved with cancer.

The sternocleidomastoid muscle is a long muscle that extends from behind the ear to the clavicle (collarbone). Turn your head to the left and stick out your chin, and you can feel this muscle in the right side of your neck stick out. Fortunately this is not an important muscle for head movement, neck, shoulder, or arm support, and there are no adverse effects from removing this muscle. However, removal can leave you with a visible depression in the tissue of your neck, resulting in one side looking flatter than the other.

The internal jugular vein is one of the major veins that drain blood flow from the head and neck. There is one on each side of the neck and the vertebral veins in addition help with blood drainage. Removal of the vein normally does not cause a noticeable effect. If the internal jugular vein is removed from both sides of the neck, a small percentage of patients may develop swelling of the head and neck that can interfere with breathing and require a temporary tracheostomy.

The spinal accessory nerve is a nerve that innervates the trapezius shoulder muscle (see **Figure 4-7 A–C**). When this nerve is injured or removed, shoulder weakness can result, causing drooping of the shoulder and inability to raise the arm above the level of the head on that side. Temporary weakness of this nerve can result after neck dissection when the nerve is saved. Shoulder weakness is still

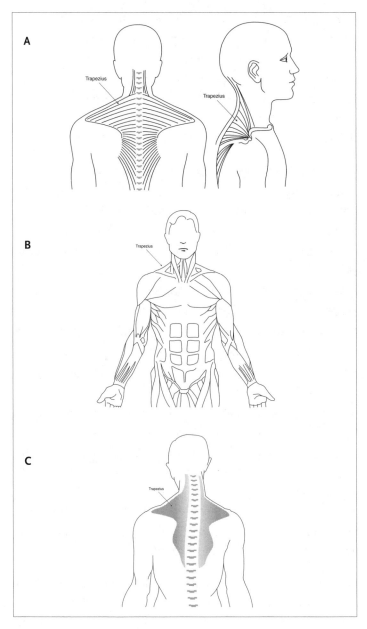

FIGURE 4-7 A–C. Trapezius muscle.

common after neck dissection even when there has been no injury to the accessory nerve. Pain limiting shoulder movement can contribute to a stiff shoulder which may not improve without therapy. A physical therapist is an important part of your recovery team if you experience shoulder weakness after surgery. Talk to your doctor about getting involved with physical therapy early after surgery.

The usual hospital stay after neck dissection alone is 1 to 3 days. Longer hospitalization is needed if additional procedures are performed at the time of neck dissection. A drain is placed under the skin at the end of surgery, and this drains any fluid that would otherwise collect under the skin flaps and interfere with healing. The drain is usually required for anywhere from 1 to 3 days after surgery on average, depending on how much fluid accumulates. Some patients are able to go home with the drain in place but the majority remain in the hospital until the drain is removed. Antibiotic ointment is applied to your incision for 2 weeks after surgery. You can clean the incision with peroxide as directed by your doctor. It takes 6 weeks before people start to feel able to resume normal function. Neck dissection is associated with a visible scar. Talk to your doctor about the types of incisions he or she may utilize. It is important to keep your scar out of the sun for 6 months after surgery to avoid darkening of the scar which makes it permanently noticeable. Purchase a zinc-oxide-based sunscreen to apply over the incision once it has healed.

Fortunately, neck dissection does not result in long-term disability for the majority of patients. Removal of the lymph nodes does not make you more susceptible to infections or cancers. We have thousands of lymph nodes all throughout our bodies. Side effects of neck dissection can include a painful scar, infection, bleeding, injury to nerves that move the shoulder, lip, and tongue, and shoulder/neck stiffness and lymphedema. Depending on the extent of your surgery, it can take 3 to 6 months for the strength in your shoulder to improve. Be patient and don't give up! If you keep the motion in your shoulder, the strength will recover more quickly. If you have had previous radiation, or are going to have radiation post-operatively, fibrosis or stiffening of the tissue is common and can affect the deeper muscles involved with swallowing. Talk to your doctor about getting involved with physical therapy early after surgery. Shoulder motion exercises can start as soon as the neck drain is removed, and, more importantly, begin meeting with a speech therapist for swallowing therapy before fibrosis occurs.

LYMPHEDEMA

It is common after neck surgery to have some swelling in your face and jaw. This swelling usually goes away after 2 to 3 weeks. If the swelling does not get better or you feel it is getting worse, you could be developing lymphedema. Lymphedema symptoms include swelling that is worse in the morning and gets better toward the end of the day and a feeling of tightness or heaviness in the face and neck. Lymphedema can be effectively treated by a specially trained physical therapist. Let your doctor know if you are having problems with swelling so you can arrange treatment as soon as possible. The following will help you reduce your risk of lymphedema:

- Keep the skin on your face and neck clean and dry.

- Use a moisturizer to prevent dry skin.

- Use a sunscreen to avoid sunburns.

- Use an electric razor to avoid cutting your face during shaving.

- If you do get a cut, wash it with soap and water and apply a triple antibiotic ointment.

- Avoid excessive heat, especially when bathing, since heat can make swelling worse.

- Use insect repellent to avoid insect stings and bites when outside, especially in the evening.

- Wear loose-fitting clothing.

XEROSTOMIA

Dry mouth is a common side effect after radiation and sometimes after surgery. If your saliva glands were removed or radiated, you may experience dry mouth or changes in saliva production after treatment. These changes are permanent. Medications are available to increase saliva production after treatment but the most important thing is to make sure your mouth is clean, kept moist, and lubricated. Drinking plenty of water is important to replace the saliva your mouth no longer makes. We make up to 1½ liters of saliva a day, which is important in lubricating the mouth and throat and helps with swallowing, as well as protecting our teeth. After radiation, you will still produce some mucous but it will be thick and sticky. It can interfere with swallowing and in severe cases, can result in mucous plugs in the airway which can be life-threatening. The most important thing you can do is be meticulous about oral hygiene, and carry plenty of water with you at all times.

Biotene® and MouthKote® are two brands of mouth care products specifically designed for people with dry mouth. They also make a topical artificial saliva that some people find useful.

Remember that xerostomia can speed up cavity development. If you have xerostomia from radiation, it is very important to make sure you have a fluoride tray to wear at least once a day to provide additional fluoride to your teeth, as well as seeing your dentist every 3 months for a cleaning. If you have had radiation therapy, remember to talk to your cancer doctor before undergoing any dental surgery as the risk of jaw complications is increased after radiation and may be minimized with hyperbaric oxygen and antibiotics.

There are certain foods and liquids which tend to worsen dry mouth or create discomfort due to dry mouth, including caffeine, alcohol, spicy foods, carbonated beverages, and foods with high acidic content. Many patients will need to avoid these foods indefinitely. This varies for each person.

MUCOSITIS

Mucositis is a common side effect of radiation, particularly when radiation is combined with chemotherapy. It results from the acute inflammation that radiation and chemotherapy cause. These treatments are targeted at killing rapidly growing cells (your cancer). The cells lining your mouth also grow quickly (as the lining of your mouth is constantly replacing itself) and are affected by the treatment. Your mouth and throat can become inflamed and raw. Your doctor will prescribe mouth rinses that contain a topical anesthetic, an anti-inflammatory agent and a coating agent to help treat the pain and soreness associated with mucositis. Sometimes an antifungal medication is used as well.

The midpoint of radiation (halfway through treatment) is a low point for many patients, when mucositis becomes most severe. It *does* get better. It is important to maintain your nutrition and stay adequately hydrated during this time. Use a humidifier in the bedroom to minimize dryness at night when you are not drinking.

SPEECH AND SWALLOWING THERAPY

The role of speech and swallowing therapy is very important in your cancer treatment plan. Cancer treatment is aimed at getting rid of the cancer and often comes at a cost of speech and swallowing function. We know these are functions that are critical for your emotional and physical well-being long after the cancer has left your body. Your doctor will refer you to meet with a speech therapist prior to starting treatment. They can counsel you as to what to expect if you are going to have surgery or a tracheostomy or stoma as part of your treatment. They will actively help you to regain your speech ability if part of your tongue or larynx is surgically removed. Even non-surgical treatment negatively affects your swallowing, and it is very important that you have a care team that recognizes and deals with this major side effect of cancer treatment.

In the case of surgery, swallowing problems can arise when important parts of the swallowing system are removed. You may notice symptoms that include difficulty with chewing, trouble moving the food from your mouth to your throat, difficulty keeping the food from spilling out of your mouth, food feeling stuck in your mouth or throat, food or liquid going up into your nose, or coughing on food/liquid when things go down the wrong way. All of these symptoms should be evaluated by the speech-language pathologist. Treatment may include changing the texture of your foods, using special feeding devices, using different postures when eating, and specific swallowing exercises to improve the way the swallowing system is working. If you have any of these symptoms, you should consult with a speech-language pathologist for further evaluation.

With radiation or chemoradiation, the structures of the swallowing system are left in place: however, sometimes they do not work as well as they did before treatment. Tissues and muscles may stiffen during radiation. When this happens, they cannot move as well as they used to. This may lead to food and pills getting stuck in your throat or food or liquids going down the wrong pipe. Recent research has shown that exercises and eating by mouth during radiation can help prevent these problems from happening. You should meet with a speech-language pathologist before your treatment begins to learn exercises which can help prevent swallowing problems after treatment is completed.

Another swallowing problem that can happen after radiation is narrowing of the food pipe, also known as an esophageal stricture. When this happens, food and sometimes liquids will build up in your food pipe instead of going down easily. You might experience food or liquid coming up after a meal or a sensation of food sticking in your throat or chest if you have an esophageal stricture. A stricture can be found during a special X-ray test called a barium swallow. If you have a stricture, this can be stretched during a simple surgical procedure performed by your head and neck surgeon or a gastroenterologist.

SPEECH AND VOICE PROBLEMS

Because of the location of tumors in the mouth, throat, and voice box, your speech and voice may also change as a result of the tumor or treatment. Speech refers to the formation of sounds in your mouth, and voice refers to the sound which comes from your voice box. The speech-language pathologist can help to evaluate and provide any treatment for issues related to speech or voice.

Surgery or radiation targeting tumors of the tongue, jaw, and palate are most likely to result in trouble forming speech sounds. Things you may notice include slurring of your speech, difficulty making certain sounds, and people having difficulty understanding you. Based upon the location and size of your tumor, the speech pathologist can give you some idea of what to expect after surgery. Treatments after your surgery or radiation may include exercises, prosthetic devices, or different ways to compensate. If you are having radiation to the mouth area, it is important to complete range of motion exercises during treatment to reduce stiffening of the muscles during treatment. The speech pathologist can guide you to the most beneficial exercises.

If you are being treated for cancer of the voice box (larynx), you may have issues with your voice that range from very minimal to total loss of the voice due to total laryngectomy. More mild problems may include reduction in the pitch range of your voice, mild hoarseness, reduced loudness, and a sense of increased effort to produce voice. Again, the speech pathologist is instrumental in evaluating the types of difficulties you are having and helping to find solutions. Voice therapy may include exercises to stretch and strengthen the muscles of the voice box, making environmental changes to improve the health of your voice box, and use of compensations such as personal voice amplifiers. If part or all of the voice box is removed, surgical procedures or prosthetic devices may be required to help you maintain communication. You should meet with the speech pathologist before treatment to discuss your individual voice needs and to establish what types of treatment may be necessary.

SUPPORTIVE CARE

It is very common for head and neck cancer patients to ask "why me?" and to become concerned about the changes in appearance and voice. There are often worries about how friends and family will react and whether or not you will be able to return to a normal life. These are normal reactions and there are many ways you can help in your own recovery.

Know what is happening to you. Discuss your concerns with your doctor or nurse. Ask questions. The health care team is concerned about your reactions and is your best source of information. Share your feelings with family and friends. Do not be afraid or embarrassed to talk with family and friends.

Attend support group meetings. Get to know how other head and neck cancer patients and their families are coping. Other people have met the same challenges you are now facing. You can also ask your doctor, nurse, or speech pathologist to meet someone who has had a similar cancer and treatment. Local and national support groups exist for head and neck cancer. Some groups are specific for total laryngectomy patients. Most support groups today are very informative and provide excellent resources for patients and families dealing with a variety of changes after treatment. There are also online support groups and web sites available. Be sure to ask your doctor or health care team for a reference to be sure you attend the right group for you.

See Chapter 11 for more information about head and neck cancer support groups.

We encourage patients to complete the following information and keep it handy.

My Family Doctor _____

My Surgeon _____

Rescue Squad _____

Home Care Company _____

Equipment:

Tracheostomy/Laryngectomy Tube (name and size) _____

_____

Suction Catheter and Size _____

Humidifier and Oxygen _____

Speaking Method _____

Other Numbers:

_____

_____

_____

FIGURE 4-8. Important numbers and information.

Please be sure that you have the following at the home where you'll be staying after your surgery:

Electric service and outlets for equipment	☐
Stairs with railings	☐
Working phone service	☐
No throw rugs	☐
Working refrigerator	☐
Adequate heat/ventilation	☐
Running water available (hot water)	☐
Working smoke detector	☐
Main bathroom/bedroom on same floor	☐
Easy access to home entrance	☐

Other_____

_____

_____

_____

_____

FIGURE 4-9. Home/environment safety checklist.

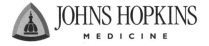

CHAPTER 5

JOHNS HOPKINS
M E D I C I N E

STRAIGHT TALK— COMMUNICATION WITH FAMILY, FRIENDS, AND COWORKERS

Heather M. Starmer, MA, MS, CCC-SLP

Dealing with cancer is complex, complicated, and difficult to talk about. It is often very hard to communicate to close family and friends what is happening to you or how you are coping. Most people also find it awkward, embarrassing, or even painful to discuss their illness. Family roles and routines may change. You may not be able to do all that you used to do. You may want to be independent but are afraid that you will become a burden to your loved ones. All these concerns or anxieties are normal, but cancer not only affects the people who have been diagnosed but everyone who cares about them. Protecting loved ones or hiding your own fears expends energy that could be channeled toward getting healthy and fighting your disease.

When you keep your family and friends informed of how you feel, both emotionally and physically, they will be able to understand your challenges, provide support, and assist you in making informed decisions. The more informed your loved ones are, the more comfortable they will be in carrying out your wishes and offering appropriate help.

SHARING YOUR CANCER DIAGNOSIS

You will most likely have many different emotions as you learn more about your diagnosis and begin to think about treatment decisions. The first step is to admit to yourself how you feel. Only you can decide when to talk to your friends and family about having cancer. Most people need and want to talk to someone. Sometimes, telling those close to you helps you to begin to take in the reality of your situation. Others find that by talking, they begin to solve problems and think about other issues that need to be sorted out.

You might give some thought to how much you wish to share about your diagnosis. You may want to explain what kind of cancer you have, which treatments you might need, and what your prognosis is. You may find it helpful to start by making a list of people who you want to tell about your cancer in person. People are very sobered by the news that someone has cancer. You may want to reassure them that you will do what is necessary to fight the cancer and would like to have their support and encouragement.

Think about which topics are too sensitive for you to talk about yet. Plan a response that is acceptable to you, and once you have shared what you wish to share, be prepared to politely end or change the conversation.

JUGGLING WITH UNEXPECTED FEELINGS

Even in the most loving families, members occasionally feel resentment when one member is ill and cannot maintain the same responsibilities for a while. This is especially true when the situation lasts for a long time. Whether they do so openly or not, family members may express anger toward you because their lives are suddenly disrupted. While you may be the only available target for such anger, keep in mind that the situation, not you, is at fault.

Though this kind of anger can be confusing and frustrating for everyone, it is a common response to a major life change. Sometimes you and your loved ones will feel out of step with each other. This may be upsetting, but remember people react differently to stressful situations. People's experiences and personalities affect how they will react to problems. Some family members may become more absorbed in work, some may become overly involved in your treatment or personal life, and others may engage in activities outside the home. The best thing you can do for each other is to be honest about what you are feeling. Fears about the future and feelings of guilt, resentment, and rage are often less frightening when you share them with others, and doing so can help all of you in the healing process.

DISCUSSING YOUR FEARS

Most people, after hearing your announcement, will be curious about the next step. They may wonder where and when you will have surgery. They may want to know if you will be undergoing radiation and/or chemotherapy. Answer their questions as best as you can, but keep in mind that "I don't know right now" or "I'm still in too much shock to think about that" are good answers.

Generally, however, discussing fears or concerns can put them into perspective. You may only realize your own feelings when someone else asks the question. Once your fears and those of your loved ones are out in the open, they can stop growing uncontrollably and causing more misconceptions. Although it may be hard to do, discussing how you are all coping with your diagnosis will make it easier to work together and make plans for the future.

FINDING YOUR OWN VOICE

If you and your family avoid talking about certain personal issues, remember that it is okay not to open up completely to everyone. This might be a good time, though, to start to work slowly on becoming more expressive with those dear to you. If you do not feel comfortable doing this, you may want to find a support group or a mental health counselor to help you. Your support group or counselor will be there for you at a regular time set aside for you to focus on your concerns and issues. Other patients prefer workshops, peer groups, or religious support. Try different things until you find what works for you. When you keep others involved and informed about your illness, it helps ease your burden.

You also may have friends or family members who tell you to "cheer up" when you tell them about your sadness or fears. It is fine to ask them gently if they would be willing just to listen, without judgment or advice. Sometimes you just have to take a couple of deep breaths and say calmly, "Thank you so much for your concern, but I need to focus on something else today." Remember, this is your illness, and it is your decision whether or not you choose to discuss it.

Some people are unable to listen, not because of you, but because of their own experiences or their own sadness. When you feel that you are pressured, you might ask a family member or friend to be your spokesperson. It can be emotionally exhausting to repeat the details of your illness to everyone who is concerned about you. This might be a good time as well to start a journal or diary if you do not already have one. There are web sites and blogs designed for cancer patients and families where they can update medical information daily without having to talk on the phone for hours about what is going on. Others send out group emails to update their concerned loved ones whenever something changes. The important thing is to find something that works for you.

TALKING WITH YOUNG CHILDREN ABOUT YOUR CANCER

Toddlers and preschoolers are very dependent upon their parents, and, as a result, are quick to notice stress or tension in the home. Don't assume that their age prevents them from feeling your stress. Though toddlers and preschoolers won't understand what cancer is, you can let them know that you are sick and that the doctors are going to work very hard to make you better. Your young child may be worried that you will go away like other relatives who have passed on. Though you may not be able to assure them this will not happen to you, acknowledging their fears may be critical to their well-being. They may also feel as though something they did caused you to be ill. It is important to reassure the child that your illness is not their fault. It is also a good idea to tell your child that sometimes you will feel sad or tired and that this is also not their fault. Let them know it is okay for them to be sad and that they can talk to you or your spouse any time they are feeling sad. Try to maintain family routines as much as is possible.

Wait until the initial wave of strong emotions has passed before telling the children in your life. Cancer is often an unfamiliar concept to them. Do not overwhelm them with too much information. They tend to understand concrete ideas and make broad generalizations, yet how they react to upsetting news depends a lot on how the adults are handling it. Adults, for instance, often want to protect their children from their fears, frustrations, and worries. However, if children are not given an honest explanation of the situation, they are likely to draw inaccurate, distressing conclusions as their imagination fills in the gaps.

When talking to children about cancer, you should give them simple yet truthful details that they will understand. How much they need to know and can handle depends on the children's age and level of maturity. Tell them a small amount of information in words that are easy for them to comprehend. Then give them both time to grasp the information and an opportunity to ask questions. Occasionally, children wrongly believe that they are to blame for their parent's or grandparent's illness. Others worry that they can "catch" cancer, that everyone dies from it, or that the other parent will get it. Kids usually will not express this, so it is a good idea to relieve some of these fears.

Many parents choose to wait to tell their children until after they've seen the doctors and know the treatment plans. It is important to remember that some treatments for head and neck cancer may alter your physical appearance, and it is important to ready your children or grandchildren for that possibility. For example, if the child has never seen you without a beard, it is a good idea to shave the beard before surgery so that they can get used to one change at a time. Your communication may also be impacted by your treatment, particularly if you have surgery. Knowing in advance what your limitations may be and discussing this with your children will help them in adapting when the time comes. If you will require some sort of communication device after surgery, you may consider introducing the device to your child before your surgery.

Many children also try to behave like adults so life will be easier for their parents. They may be asked to do extra chores or be on their best behavior if people other than their parents are helping to care for them. They may question or even resent a lack of attention. They may focus on death or separation. It is important to try and maintain a "normal" routine and lifestyle for children, but they need to be prepared for the changes that will happen in the family. If appropriate, you may also wish to have a social worker or school psychologist talk with your child. They may know of support groups for children in your area or offer a new source of support that is outside of your own family.

Parents should not pretend that there is nothing to worry about. It is okay if your children see you crying from time to time. The key is to make your children realize that cancer is a serious—but not a hopeless—disease. Children should be encouraged to express all of their feelings—good and bad. They may wish to show their feelings through painting, writing, or puppets. Be prepared overall to reassure your children of your love, even if you are in the hospital or feeling sick.

Try to talk about your treatment in a positive way if possible, rather than dwelling on all the distressing or negative side effects. If you are going to lose your hair from chemotherapy, for instance, tell your children so they will not be afraid when it happens. If you will be in the hospital, children need to know where, for how long, what is going to happen, whether they can visit or at least call, and who will take care of them. Children should be told that mom or dad might be a bit "grouchy" or irritable during treatment, but that it is not their fault.

Depending on the age and maturity level of the child, it may be worth considering attending a support group for patients with head and neck cancer before your treatment. In addition, many major cancer centers will offer educational programs for children to introduce them to the hospital and treatments to help reduce their fears and anxieties regarding the unknown. If your child has many questions about your treatment, attending such a program may help to reduce their fears and uncertainty.

TALKING WITH OLDER CHILDREN AND TEENS

If your children are older, they may be anxious or even angry about how this will impact them. Teens often view the world as revolving around them, and they may feel resentful about how changes in routine will impact them. These natural teen responses can be magnified by their fear of losing a parent. As every child is different, it is important to know where they are coming from mentally and emotionally. Keeping communication lines open is critical, particularly for children in this age group. You will have to decide who will tell the kids and when, but also how much detail you want to share with them and at what intervals. Their knowledge of cancer in general may be to associate it with death. Ask your child what they know about cancer and then provide them with details at their level. Reassure them honestly about your treatment and prognosis.

Teens may be particularly resentful when asked to help out around the house. There is some evidence that teens are unable to psychologically cope with the responsibility of filling a parent's role during such times of upheaval. Teens may then feel guilty about their feelings of resentment, further compounding an unfortunate situation. Find ways for the older child to contribute to the family while maintaining typical roles and boundaries as much as possible. Explain to them that you may need extra help around the house for a while, but also take steps to show balance between family responsibilities and normal teenage lifestyles. Discuss how the family will work to balance responsibilities.

TELLING YOUR ADULT CHILDREN AND PARENTS

Even adult children worry that their parents will die or become sick. When they learn that you have cancer, adult children may realize how important you are to them. They may experience guilt if they have not been that close. They may feel horrible if they cannot spend a lot of time with you because they live far away or have employment obligations. Your relationship with your adult children will probably change now that you have cancer, and you should include them when talking about your treatment.

You should also decide how much to tell your parents about your cancer. Your decision may depend on how well your parents can understand and cope with the news. If your parents are in good health, think about talking with them about your cancer. You may need extra help caring for your parents or you may need assistance only during your treatment. Mothers in particular are used to making everything better for their children and may want to try to control the situation for you. They may be frustrated when they can't guide or control your treatment and recovery. They will need to be given constructive ways to help because no matter what, they will want to help you—even if you feel you don't need it. Mothers can fill an important role in the home if there are children to care for.

Other family members will also have unique relationships that need to be considered. Fathers, like mothers, may have difficulty accepting the illness of their child and may need special consideration. Siblings may also feel great grief and concern for your well-being. Having them assist with information gathering can help engage them in your treatment and empower them with information that will help both of you. Family can also be critical for providing and coordinating assistance during your treatment. Remember that every offer for assistance is genuine. Be ready to accept assistance. Keep your family members informed of how you are doing as treatment progresses. Remember, this is a disease that affects the entire family. The feelings of fear and apprehension you have are shared by many.

INFORMING YOUR FRIENDS

The decision to discuss your diagnosis with friends is yours alone. However, it is usually best to be honest about your cancer with people close to you. Keeping it a secret can cause you more stress at a time when you could use the support of others. Before you talk to others about your illness, think through your own feelings, your reasons for telling them, and your expectations of them. Often, people do not know what to say, which makes them feel awkward and uncomfortable. They might be frightened about the possibility of losing you. They may feel that it is easier to say nothing because they are afraid of saying the wrong thing. They may withdraw or distance themselves. Some may become overly considerate or intrusive. Most likely, your friends will want to help you, but they may be uncertain how. Allow friends and family to help you. Be specific as this makes it easier for them to think that they are included in your life.

Once people have had time to adjust to the news, do not be afraid to communicate to them what is happening with you. Explain what kind of cancer you have and the treatments you will need. Tell them that cancer is not a death sentence, nor is it contagious. Find out what they think and how they feel, and try to answer their questions. Try to be direct with others and express your needs and feelings openly. It is generally more stressful to hide emotions than to express them, and sharing with other people can be helpful both to you and those close to you.

People will undoubtedly ask what they can do to help you. It may be helpful to identify a coordinator early on who can delegate tasks to well-doers. Among the many things people can do are:

- Drive you to appointments
- Drive your children to school and events
- Run errands
- Make meals for your freezer
- Baby-sit
- Help with the housework
- Add you to prayer lists at church.

Remember that these people want to do something to help and would not offer if they did not sincerely want to provide assistance. One day, perhaps you will be able to reciprocate and help in a crisis as well.

On the other hand, some friends may avoid calling you after they hear the news. It isn't that they don't care; it's more likely that they don't know what to say. Let them know that even though the diagnosis is upsetting to hear, you need their support. Remember that support from others is an important part of your treatment plan for you and your family.

BALANCING NEW RELATIONSHIPS

The same ideas apply to people who are single, but you may feel unsure how and when to talk about having cancer if you are single or if you are just starting to date someone. Trust yourself to be the judge of the best time to share this part of your life with someone. You may want to talk about it very early in a relationship or you might wish to wait until you feel a closer bond with the person. You may find it helps to practice what you will say with a friend before sharing with your new partner.

For single men or women without supportive family members nearby, it may be even more important to let close friends know about your cancer and treatment. You may not feel okay going home alone after surgery or chemotherapy. You may need someone you can call if you have trouble during the night. Remember that your friends want to assist you, and by communicating what you need, you can facilitate more supportive and rewarding relationships.

LETTING YOUR BOSSES AND COWORKERS KNOW

It is common to be concerned about maintaining your job after treatment. Fortunately, the American Disabilities Act (ADA) provides some job protection. You should be able to work with your boss on a schedule that will meet your medical needs as well as the needs of your employer. You are not actually required to tell your boss you have cancer.

It is fine to explain that you are under doctor's care that will require you to miss time from work. Most individuals will tell their boss that they have been diagnosed with cancer and will be undergoing whatever treatments have been recommended. You are not responsible to provide information about your prognosis.

As with friends and family, deciding what to tell coworkers can be difficult. Many people will choose to inform coworkers in vague terms rather than providing full details of their treatment plan. There are advantages to letting key people know as you will more than likely require some time off for treatment. Again, this is your personal business and whatever feels right in your situation is the best answer. As with family, offers of assistance from friends and coworkers are typically genuine and it is beneficial for you as well as the helpers to involve them as needed.

During and after treatment, the need to update people on your situation can be a job in and of itself. You may want to assign someone to be the "information center" to provide all announcements about how you are doing, what treatment you are having, pathology results, and so on. There are also a number of online resources for posting such information such as www.caringbridge.com, a free, personalized web site that will keep friends and family informed during difficult times. The web site includes a patient care journal to update family and friends, photo gallery, and guest book where visitors can post messages of support and encouragement. Email is another good way to make sure that everyone is receiving the same information at the same time and in the same manner. Have one of your family or friends who want to help gather important email addresses and enlist someone to send out broadcast emails to everyone at once. You will find such options to be a great time saver to help reduce the burden on you and ensure consistency in the information being provided. It also helps prevent hurt feelings and discontent if one person finds out you called someone else first.

SUMMING UP—SHARING YOUR THOUGHTS AND FEELINGS ABOUT CANCER

Cancer is hard to deal with all alone. It can rob people of a sense of control over their lives. Although talking about your cancer can be hard at first, most patients find that being honest and open about their cancer and the problems that arise helps them to handle the changes that their disease causes.

Remember the following as you begin communication about your cancer:

- Choose a good listener.
- Select an appropriate time to share.
- Recognize your own anger or frustrations.
- Be honest about your emotions.
- Utilize additional community resources if feeling overwhelmed.

Remember that support from others is an important part of your treatment plan for you and your family. Do not be afraid to seek that support during this most critical time.

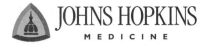

CHAPTER 6

MAINTAINING BALANCE—WORK AND LIFE DURING TREATMENT

Erin J. Blume, BS, RHIA
Carol S. Maragos, MSN, CRNP, CNOR

HELPFUL HINTS ON HOW TO PLAN CARE AND MINIMIZE DISRUPTIONS IN YOUR LIFE

Having major surgery and going through radiation and/ or chemotherapy can thoroughly disrupt your life. Head and neck cancer treatment may alter roles, play havoc with schedules, and create additional stress for the patient, other family members, and other relationships during this time. It is inevitable, but certain things can be done to prevent major chaos.

Many people may ask what they can do for you during this time. Often, patients feel uncomfortable asking for help, especially head and neck cancer patients. Don't be afraid to accept this help. Designate someone to coordinate the help that is offered. For example, a family or friend can be the person to go to when others offer their help. This person can:

- Answer phone calls, read the email messages, and email a regular health update to family and friends.

- Prepare a list of what you need to have done. This can include running errands to the grocery store, post office, cleaners, taking the children to birthday parties, athletic events, doing laundry, cleaning your house, etc.

- Coordinate meals (for example, when you want them delivered) so that you have adequate refrigerator or freezer space.

- Coordinate hospital visiting time so that you are not bombarded with visitors.

Patients with children especially may experience a variety of role changes. Daddy may be putting young children to bed because mommy doesn't feel well tonight. Older children may be asked to help with meal preparation or laundry. It's important for you and your family to talk about your schedules and how treatment needs will impact them. Design a new schedule to best meet your needs and those of your loved ones—with as little change as possible.

Try to maintain your children's routines as much as possible. Change creates stress no matter what the age. Even an infant who is fed an hour later than usual expresses feelings about his altered schedule. Let your children know in advance if there will be a change in their routine. Keep children informed about what is happening related to treatment. Encourage them to help and play an active role in the treatment. Have younger children (ages 6 to 12) go with you to the hospital when you go to one of your appointments to better understand what is happening. Ask them how they picture the treatment destroying any bad cells. Have them draw pictures to cheer you up and open your get-well cards you receive in the mail. Explain why you don't feel well and the importance of playing quietly on certain days after treatment. Let young children know that they can't catch head and neck cancer and also that they aren't in any way the cause of it.

In preparation for surgery, request to meet with an otolaryngology nurse or speech therapist for some pre-operative teaching. You will want to know in advance if you will be having a tracheostomy tube or laryngeal stoma, a feeding tube, any drains in place, how long you will be out of commission from doing your routine activities, what clothing will be best to wear post-op, when you will be allowed to resume driving, etc.

If you are scheduled to have chemotherapy and/or radiation, make a chart of when your treatments will be. Decide if you want someone to go with you for radiation or chemotherapy treatments or not. You will be in the chemotherapy infusion center for several hours, so plan accordingly. The day needs to be as laid back as possible for you. Depending on who is available to help and what your schedules end up being, you may decide that chemo days are "pizza night" for the kids or to pull the casserole your neighbor made out of the freezer.

For radiation, consider scheduling it at the very beginning of the day or end of the day rather than in the middle. Since this treatment is daily, you will want it to cause as little disruption to your daily routine as possible. Most radiation facilities have patients in and out in less than 30 minutes.

CONTINUING WORK

If your doctor has cleared you for work, you may want to work while undergoing head and neck cancer treatment. Time missed from work is usually minimal, if planned out relatively well. Sit down with your boss and plan out a schedule that works for both of you. There may be some days you only work half a day because you are getting chemotherapy in the afternoon then taking off the following day. During radiation you may be coming in an hour later to work or leaving 30 minutes early to get to your daily radiation appointment. You may need to utilize the family medical leave act protocol for time off. If you work around small children, though, especially toddlers, this may be problematic during chemotherapy because your risk of getting an infection is increased during this time.

DENTAL HEALTH

Schedule an appointment with your dentist at least 2 weeks prior to receiving treatment so that they can thoroughly examine your teeth. Infected or decaying teeth will need to be removed to prevent serious infections later (see Chapter 3). While you are receiving radiation, you will need to apply fluoride treatments daily, take meticulous care of your mouth and teeth, and eat healthy.

WHEN I MIGHT EXPECT TO NOT FEEL WELL

If you will be receiving chemotherapy, you may experience GI side effects about 16 to 48 hours after the completion of the infusion of the chemotherapy drugs. Request anti-nausea meds in advance so you can head off GI symptoms before they happen.

Depending on the type of chemotherapy you receive, hair loss usually happens between day 10 and day 14 after the first cycle of chemotherapy treatment. If you want to be proactive, consider cutting your hair short or even doing your own buzz cut prior to your hair falling out on its own. A "coming out" party for your hair is fun for kids to do for you. Friends and family bring you various head coverings, such as turbans, hats, etc., and your kids can make you some funny ones for wearing in the privacy of your own home.

In addition to the side effects mentioned, you will have a lower resistance to infection. You may have sores in your mouth and on the lips, loss of appetite, diarrhea, skin rash, joint pain, or numbness/tingling in your hands and feet.

When you are undergoing radiation treatments, anticipate feeling fine for about the first 2 weeks of radiation. At this point in time you may notice increased fatigue. This is because radiation is cumulative. Even after the radiation sessions are completed, you will continue to experience side effects. Give yourself extra time to rest at night and even a cat nap in the middle of the day if possible. Other side effects include dry mouth (xerostomia), mouth ulcers (mucositis), tooth decay, infection, skin redness, irritation and skin hardness (fibrosis), difficulty swallowing (dysphagia), a stiff jaw (trismus), changes in the way food tastes, changes in the way that dentures fit, and changes to your voice. There are many aids that can help with the dry mouth and mucositis, including prescription medications. Please talk with your oncologist and/or oncology nurse for a list of these products and/or prescriptions. You will need to consume plenty of fluids, preferably water, to prevent dehydration.

INFECTION PREVENTION

There will be certain days that it will be anticipated that your white blood cells will go down in response to receiving chemotherapy and/or radiation. These are days you are more vulnerable to getting a cold, flu, or other form of infection. You want to avoid being in the presence of youngsters since they can be sick but don't act like they are. Wearing a mask is beneficial if you can't avoid being around children in a closed environment. If you need to travel by air while undergoing chemotherapy and/or radiation, wear a mask to reduce risk of exposure. Wash your hands with soap and water or hand gel often, and have your family and visitors do the same. Hand washing is the best thing that you can do to prevent getting sick. Eating a balanced diet, rich in fruits and vegetables, helps to improve your immune system. Getting a flu shot before you start treatment is advisable too. If you are receiving treatment in the winter, be sure to bundle yourself up when going outdoors. Your mission is to be healthy during your treatments and reduce risk of exposure to infection as much as possible. The nurse working with you during your treatments can mark on your chart the days that you will be particularly vulnerable to infection. Your blood will be periodically drawn to assess how your body's immune system is responding to the treatments and whether any medicines to boost your white blood cells need to be given.

Doing as much as you can to optimize your physical and emotional health during treatment maximizes your chances of calling yourself a survivor in the not too distant future.

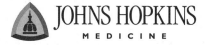

CHAPTER 7

SURVIVING CANCER— RE-ENGAGING IN MIND AND BODY HEALTH AFTER TREATMENT

Kimberly Webster, MA, MS, CCC-SLP
Carol S. Maragos, MSN, CRNP, CNOR

SURVIVORSHIP

When do you consider yourself a survivor? The most common definition is actually the moment you are diagnosed and have chosen to embark on treatment. Some people though don't consider themselves survivors until treatment is completed. You are among an elite group. When you finish your treatment, however, rather than feeling like celebrating you may feel like you fell off a cliff. This is not an unusual reaction either. You've been so focused on actively fighting this disease that when it's time to stop, you feel a sense of loss. You may be fearful, too, that you haven't done enough, or that there isn't additional treatment to continue to take as a means of preventing recurrence.

Fear of recurrence remains the biggest issue that survivors have to deal with today. Though the majority of patients won't face recurrence of this disease, it can be hard to learn to trust your body again. Staying in the know about the latest research that has been published about head and neck cancer is helpful and empowering. Taking measures to regain emotional balance is wise too. Ask your health care providers for a list of support groups who may help with this purpose (many of these are listed in Chapter 11). Get involved with your local support group.

COUNSELING

If your doctor or nurse recommends that you consider seeing a counselor, don't feel like you have failed at getting yourself back on track. It's hard. Many patients would benefit from seeing a therapist after treatment to help them physically and emotionally. Sometimes we just need a professional sounding board to hear our hidden thoughts and fears and help us gain perspective about what and what not to worry about. You want to regain control over your life. This can take assistance from others who are professionally trained. Diagnosis and treatment of head and neck cancer can be a life-altering experience. There is no operator's manual for this experience. Talk with other survivors, too, so that you can realize that what you are experiencing is the norm and not the exception.

MANAGING LONG-TERM SIDE EFFECTS OF TREATMENT

It would be great if at the time treatment ended, all the side effects associated with it ended too, but this is not the case. You may be dealing with residual side effects of fatigue, difficulty with swallowing, mouth dryness and/or ulcers, arm weakness, peripheral neuropathy, difficulty concentrating, or other unpleasantness. Give your body time to heal and adjust. Some side effects like fatigue can linger for 1 year. Don't expect to feel back to yourself the week treatments end. There is a period of psychological and physical adjustment, similar to becoming pregnant and 9 months later giving birth. Your body needs time. Allow it this time. See Chapters 3 and 4 for management of side effects.

LIVING A HEALTHIER LIFESTYLE

Taking charge of your health and psychological well-being should be a priority for you now and has proven survival benefits. Here are some helpful ways to accomplish this and feel good doing it.

NUTRITION

It is important to take in a high-quality nutritional diet so that you will continue to heal. Now is not the time to try to lose weight. If you are able to eat by mouth, eat a healthy diet that consists of fruits, vegetables, whole grains, and protein. Reduce the amount of red meat and fat in your diet. If you are taking nutrition through a feeding tube, take in the amount that was prescribed for you. If you are unable to use the recommended amount of cans, contact your primary care physician or nutritionist. Your body needs nutrients to continue to heal.

EXERCISE

This is another way to help reduce risk of recurrence. This doesn't mean you need to become a marathon runner and bench press 400 pounds at the gym. It does mean finding an exercise program that works for you, that you can commit to, and makes you feel good. If you enjoy the exercise program, do it in an environment that makes you feel comfortable, feel better after you do it, and is something you are able to stick with, then it's a winner for you. Power walking is one of those options to consider. Walking three times a week for an hour will suffice, as will working out three times a week if approved by your doctor. Exercising with a friend usually makes it more enjoyable and helps you to stick to it because you have a buddy supporting you.

STRESS

Emotional turmoil affects our immune system, and our immune system needs to be in good shape to fight cancer cells and prevent cancer cells from growing. You will be expected to resume your chaotic life, including family responsibilities and work duties. That can be quite stressful. You may need to reassess how you react to stressful situations. Head and neck cancer can teach us that we really don't have to sweat the small stuff. Making time for you is important, including when treatment is completed. Put things into perspective before reacting to them. Ask yourself: "Is it really a crisis if my mother-in-law comes over and I haven't dusted or vacuumed the floors?" You have been through much bigger and more significant events. Learning deep breathing techniques, taking a yoga class, or doing other forms of relaxation therapy can be helpful to you in reducing stress and keeping life in perspective.

AVOID SMOKE AND ALCOHOL

This includes secondary smoke. If you have a friend who smokes, remind him or her that if he cares about you he will take his cigarettes outside. If he refuses and still smokes around you then he isn't your friend. Limit alcohol intake to only one drink on social occasions.

SETTING NEW GOALS

You have just completed treatment that is life-altering. You have perhaps stared death in the face and survived what you thought wasn't possible to overcome. This is an ideal time to step back and reassess your life, looking at how you want to leave your mark on this earth, now realizing you are going to be around to make that mark. Some people decide they want to go back to school. Others decide they want to work part-time rather than full-time and spend more time with their family. Consider setting short-term goals and long-term goals. Some goals may be directed at living a healthier life style; others may be focused on how you want to make a difference for others who come behind you and are diagnosed with this disease. You are connected to an extraordinary group of patients who share common thoughts, dreams, and fears. Band together to make a difference or strike out on your own regarding how you want to spend the rest of your life. What you thought was important before may have little meaning now. This can be quite confusing though to those around you who were expecting things to return to "normal." You need to find your "new normal," and let your family and friends know that you are working hard to accomplish this. This experience has changed you, hopefully for the better, and life will be considered more precious and valued than it was before. You have gotten in touch with your mortality. No doubt about it. Communicate with your family and friends your thoughts. Keep a journal to record them. Journaling is very therapeutic.

SEEING THE WORLD THROUGH DIFFERENT EYES

It can be hard for the people you spend time with—to family, friends, and coworkers—because you may not seem like the same person you were before your diagnosis. Hopefully you are different in all the right ways. Mindful of how precious life is. Never taking anything for granted. Valuing relationships differently than you did before. Consider getting involved as a volunteer. One of the best ways to move forward with your experience with head and neck cancer is to help those who are diagnosed after you. By helping someone else, you help yourself psychologically because, although recovery from head and neck cancer itself may take a long time physically, emotional recovery can take a lifetime. It can and usually is life-altering in a positive way. Consider volunteering where you received your treatments or volunteer for a head and neck cancer organization that has a chapter in your area. This is very rewarding and a great way to give back as well as help others and yourself. Educate others and help promote head and neck cancer awareness in your local community. You can save other people's lives by promoting early intervention, smoking cessation, and alcohol cessation.

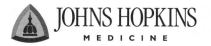

CHAPTER 8

MANAGING RISK—WHAT IF MY CANCER COMES BACK?

Christine G. Gourin, MD, FACS

R isk of recurrence is one of the biggest fears of patients who have finished treatment for head and neck cancer. Learning what to look for, when, how, and for how long is helpful. Putting your risk of recurrence into perspective is extremely important to your psychological well-being. You can't know the future, but you can take steps to make sure you are doing everything possible to avoid recurrence and catch it early if it happens.

PREVENTION AND MONITORING FOR RECURRENCE

The risk of tumor recurrence varies from patient to patient, depending on the tumor type, stage, and location. With the exception of some benign tumors, the risk is never zero. As a general rule, the 5-year cancer-free survival rates for patients with most head and neck cancers are 80% to 100% for stage 1 cancer, 60% to 80% for stage 2 cancer, 40% to 60% for stage 3, and 20% to 40% for stage 4 cancer. The risk of recurrence increases as the tumor stage increases. The exact numbers vary depending on the exact type of tumor and its location, but these rough guidelines hold true for most patients. In addition, there are some prognostic factors that may influence these numbers, such as the presence of perineural invasion (spread along nerves), extracapsular spread in lymph nodes, the risk of distant metastases for patients with stage 4 cancer, and close or positive surgical margins, all of which are associated with a higher incidence of recurrent disease. The risk of recurrence is greatest during the first 2 years following treatment. Once this milestone of time is reached, the risk of recurrence lessens considerably. For many types of head and neck cancer, the risk of recurrence approaches zero at 5 years, at which point you are considered cured.

There is a separate risk and that is the development of second primary tumors of the head and neck. Patients with squamous cell cancer, or those with a history of previous radiation therapy to the head and neck, are at risk for developing a second cancer unrelated to the first. Between 10% to 20% of patients with a history of head and neck cancer will develop a second primary cancer during their lifetime. The exact incidence varies depending on the tumor type, but patients who smoke and drink alcohol are at increased risk. The reasons for this are not clear, but it is believed that a combination of environmental and genetic factors result in the development of head and neck cancer, and those individuals who may have been successfully treated for head and neck cancer in the past are still at risk for developing a second cancer from those same factors (which still exist). Radiation-induced cancers are rare and are defined as tumors occurring in areas that have previously been treated with radiation 5 years ago or longer and are believed to result from cell damage induced by the radiation rather than being related to the former cancer.

When cancer recurs, it can recur locally—at the site of the initial primary tumor—regionally in the neck, or at distant sites, such as the lungs, liver, or bones. There are measures you can take to both lessen your risk of recurrence as well as being vigilant about follow-up examinations and being on guard for new symptoms so that if your cancer recurs, it can be detected early, which improves your chances of survival.

PREVENTION

If you smoke, now is the time to stop. The likelihood of developing head and neck cancer is greatly increased in people who smoke or drink, and people who both smoke and drink have more than three times the risk of developing cancer compared to the risk from smoking or drinking alone. You can lower that risk by quitting now. Smoking decreases the likelihood that treatment will be successful, thus increasing the risk of recurrence and increasing the risk of developing a second primary tumor. Other factors that may contribute to head and neck cancer include poor oral hygiene, poor nutrition, a weakened immune system, and oral trauma. These are factors that are within your control and you should take active steps to do everything possible to reverse these.

MONITORING FOR RECURRENCE

Your doctor will recommend scheduled follow-up visits after treatment to monitor you for recurrence or the development of a new tumor. As a general rule, patients undergo a complete head and neck evaluation by their surgeon every 1 to 2 months for the first 2 years after treatment, every 3 months for the third year, every 6 months for the fourth and fifth years, and annually thereafter. This examination will include the use of endoscopes for areas that are not easily examined with a headlight. Your doctor may order an imaging study, such as a CT or PET-CT scan, to look for tumor recurrence. Your first scan should not performed until all of the swelling and inflammation from treatment have subsided. This will take at least 3 months. Scans done before this may mistake tissue that is simply reacting to the cancer treatment for a recurrence of the cancer itself. The interval at which you will need specialized imaging studies varies depending on risk factors, tumor stage, and tumor type. For example, patients with early-stage cancer do not need a PET-CT scan, and not all types of cancers will show up on a PET-CT scan. Those studies are repeated at intervals of several months for the first 2 years in patients who are at high risk for recurrence because of advanced-stage aggressive tumor types. At a minimum, all patients should undergo an annual chest X-ray unless their tumor was benign. There are no blood tests for tumor markers that are useful in the follow-up of patients with head and neck cancer.

SYMPTOM AWARENESS

In addition to having a formal examination by your doctor, you should become tuned in to your body. If your tissues have undergone a change from treatment, become used to the feel and appearance of your mouth and your neck. Essentially, you are doing your own self-examination in between visits to your head and neck surgeon. Any new lump in the neck or sore in the mouth should be a cause for concern and warrants a visit to your head and neck surgeon. In addition, there are some other symptoms that can be associated with head and neck cancer. You need to be aware of these and if you develop any one of these symptoms, you should see your physician. Some of the more common symptoms that may be associated with head and neck cancer include:

- Ear pain, especially if only on one side

- Painful swallowing

- New difficulty swallowing

- Sore throat

- Foreign body sensation or lump in your throat

- Change in mole or new skin lesion

- Non-healing mouth ulcer

- Change in denture fit

- New voice changes (hoarseness or a muffled voice)

- Difficulty opening your mouth (trismus)

- Coughing or spitting up blood

- Weight loss

- Neck lump

- Nasal obstruction or bleeding, particularly if only on one side

Tell your doctor about other symptoms if they signal a change to you from what is normal. For example, a new chronic symptom such as low back pain that is constant and doesn't go away after several weeks, abdominal pain, or unexplained weight loss, may be a signal that cancer has developed in a distant location and may warrant further investigation.

TREATMENT OPTIONS TO MANAGE RECURRENCE

Head and neck cancer can recur locally, at the site of the initial primary tumor; regionally, referring to the lymph nodes of the neck; or distantly, in organs such as the lungs, bones, or liver. Treatment options to manage recurrence depend on 1) the type of treatment you initially had 2) the extent of the recurrence and 3) the location.

When cancer recurs locally, most of the time it is where it started or very close to the original tumor location. Cancer that recurs at the site of the initial primary tumor within 5 years of treatment is considered a recurrence of the original cancer. If more than 5 years have passed since treatment, it is usually considered to be a new primary tumor. However some tumors, such as adenoid cystic cancer, can recur 10 to 15 years after treatment. Treatment options depend on the initial type of treatment you received previously, the location, and the size of the recurrence.

If you have received radiation previously, either as initial treatment or post-operatively, more radiation is usually not an option for treatment of your recurrent cancer. In this situation surgery is your best choice, but if the recurrent tumor can not be completely removed surgically, palliative chemotherapy or reirradiation may be your only options. If surgery was part of your original treatment, then the extent and location of your recurrence factor into the decision about further treatment. Some recurrences can be treated with additional surgery. When the recurrence is advanced, either post-operative radiation or chemo-radiation is usually required. Patients with large recurrences who have not received radiation previously may be better served with radiation or chemo-radiation if the tumor is in a location where surgical treatment would be expected to result in comparable survival to non-operative treatment and surgery would result in greater functional disability than non-operative treatment. Exceptions include oral cavity tumors, some salivary gland tumors, and tumors involving bone which have a poorer response to radiation therapy. Because oral cavity tumors have better cure and control rates with surgical treatment, surgery is the preferred method of treating a recurrence unless the tumor is inoperable.

Regional recurrence refers to recurrence within the lymph nodes of the neck. Because we have hundreds of lymph nodes in the neck, most too small to see with the naked eye, this can occur in up to 10% of patients despite having undergone neck dissection. As for local recurrence, your treatment options depend upon both the type of treatment you received and the extent of the recurrent disease in the neck. If you have had previous radiation therapy, neck dissection surgery is the only curative option to manage neck recurrence. If you have not had previous radiation to the neck, then treatment depends on the extent of neck disease. Patients with limited neck involvement can be treated with neck dissection followed by post-operative radiation therapy. Patients with large bulky advanced neck disease have a high risk of distant metastases, and require chemoradiation therapy. In some cases, this may be preferable to performing neck dissection if neck disease is very advanced or is inoperable.

Inoperable disease is defined as tumor that is either 1) unresectable or 2) incurable. Before embarking on any surgical attempts to "salvage" a recurrence, your surgeon needs to determine if the cancer is resectable and if distant metastases are present. Unresectable cancer refers to cancer that invades structures such as the prevertebral muscles of the spine, the carotid artery, the base of the skull, the chest, or the brain. A tumor cannot be completely removed from these areas, and the complication rate of attempted surgery is unacceptably high. Unresectable cancer does not always mean incurable cancer; sometimes a good response is seen if chemoradiation can be used in these circumstances. Incurable disease refers to disease that has metastasized to distant sites or areas that cannot be treated conventionally with curative doses of radiation, such as brain or spinal cord involvement. In addition, extensive advanced-stage recurrent disease in patients who have previously received radiation therapy is usually incurable, as the failure rate of surgery alone for advanced disease is extremely high, and normal doses of radiation therapy or chemoradiation cannot be used. In such a case, treatment should be palliative, not curative, as treatment for curative intent will not succeed, and the risks of side effects are too great. Individuals may have lung metastases that they are unaware of because they do not have symptoms. In such a case, the use of palliative chemotherapy may make that individual feel worse, and the toxicity of treatment can outweigh any benefit. Palliative treatment is directed at relieving symptoms—not at trying to achieve a cure. Radical surgery is not indicated for incurable disease. "Debulking" surgery, trying to remove as much as possible and then treating with radiation and/or chemotherapy, has not been shown to be of any benefit and is associated with significant wound healing complications when visible tumor is left behind following surgery.

Distant metastases are considered incurable, with rare exceptions—sometimes a solitary lung metastasis can be removed. However, in most cases, distant metastases indicate that cancer has spread beyond the head and neck through the blood stream, and in most patients it is only a matter of months before new sites of distant recurrence appear. Distant metastases can be treated with palliative chemotherapy or radiation to treat symptoms when these arise by trying to shrink tumor size. If you have previously been treated with chemotherapy, the drug choices will likely be different than what was originally given to you because your tumor is probably resistant to the original drug used.

If the chance of cure with radical treatment is very small, you need to have a frank discussion with your physicians about what to expect from therapy. The effect of heroic treatment on your quality of life may be unacceptable. These are hard decisions and should be made only after careful and long discussion with your treatment team and family. These decisions are examined in greater detail in the next chapter.

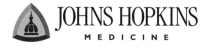

CHAPTER 9

My Cancer Isn't Curable—
What Now

Christine G. Gourin, MD, FACS

UNDERSTANDING GOALS OF TREATMENT FOR INCURABLE DISEASE

A diagnosis of incurable cancer is devastating news. We all hold onto the hope that modern medicine is capable of curing all disease, but the reality is that not all cancer is curable. It is a normal reaction to feel grief, anger, and depression. You may choose to seek a second opinion. Your doctors should not take this personally and should be supportive. The goals of treatment of incurable disease are palliative, not curative. That is, the goal becomes to control pain and manage symptoms while maintaining the best quality of life possible. It is important to have realistic expectations about treatment. Treatment options for incurable disease will not be expected to result in cure. However, you can realistically expect that treatment for incurable disease should bring you relief. There are active measures that can be taken to relieve pain and symptoms caused by your cancer, and you are in control of what treatment course you wish to pursue. There is every reason to be optimistic that you can control your quality of life for the time you have remaining.

Chemotherapy, radiation therapy, and pain management are some of the options available for patients with incurable disease. Incurable disease refers to disease that has metastasized to distant sites, cancer that involves extensive areas that cannot be treated conventionally with curative doses of radiation, such as brain or spinal cord involvement, or cancer that has recurred, is inoperable, and prior treatment limits the doses of radiation or chemoradiation that can be used. In these circumstances, additional treatment may be possible, but it is important to have realistic expectations about what treatment can accomplish. The goals of treatment are now to relieve pain and symptoms, and such treatment should maintain or improve your quality of life. In some circumstances, treatment may not be appropriate if it will worsen your quality of life by making you sick.

Treatment options for terminal disease may include chemotherapy, additional doses of radiation therapy, pain management, or hospice. The options depend on the type and location of the tumor and your previous treatment. There are some tumors that may be incurable, but patients can live for years by managing tumor growth through aggressive treatment, such as adenoid cystic carcinoma. In such cases the cancer can be managed like many other chronic diseases, such as diabetes or high blood pressure, for some years. It is important to have a frank discussion with your doctor about what to expect so you can make informed choices and plans. Pain management is the most important part of care for all patients with terminal cancer because the reality is that pain control is directly related to your quality of life. Pain can be successfully managed with medications, and most centers have pain specialists who usually have a background in anesthesia and have special expertise in the control of chronic pain. Request to meet with a pain specialist if this has not been recommended already. The goal of pain medication is to control pain while minimizing side effects. If one medication isn't working, there are other medications, alone or in combination, that can be used. Do not be concerned about becoming addicted. This is just not a real concern for most patients with terminal cancer. The need for pain medication is directly proportional to the amount of pain one is experiencing. Do not allow yourself to suffer simply to avoid a feeling of dependence on a medication. Depression can make perception of pain worse, and if depressive symptoms are severe, antidepressant therapy can be very useful.

In some circumstances, short-term relief of pain can be accomplished by using chemotherapy or radiation to shrink a tumor. Radiation can be very effective in treating bone pain from metastases. The options depend on the type of tumor and its location. If you have previously been treated with chemotherapy, your doctors will likely use different drugs than you received before as the tumor has likely become resistant to the previously used drugs. Similarly, if you have had radiation before, you may not be able to receive additional radiation. Whether or not you can receive additional radiation depends on the dose previously used and the site involved. Steroids are sometimes used to decrease swelling from tumor growth and can sometimes be of benefit.

Your physician may recommend that you undergo feeding tube placement, most commonly with a percutaneous gastrostomy tube (PEG). Head and neck cancers can interfere with swallowing, and maintaining adequate nutrition is an important part of palliative care. Weight loss can make you feel worse, and supplemental nutrition can be administered through a PEG. Anything you can put in a blender can go into a PEG. In addition, if swallowing becomes difficult, taking pain medications may also become difficult. Pain medications can be crushed or obtained in liquid form and given through the PEG. A PEG requires a minor surgical procedure by a surgeon or radiologist to insert but is preferable in the long run to a feeding tube passed through the nose, which can irritate the nose and throat if required for more than 1 to 2 weeks. It is best to have the PEG placed early if it is recommended that you consider this, rather than waiting until significant weight loss has occurred as healing problems can occur in patients who are malnourished.

Patients who are having trouble breathing because tumors involving the larynx (voice box) or throat are blocking airflow often benefit from having a tracheostomy tube placed early. Shortness of breath is the single hardest symptom for a patient to deal with and the hardest to relieve. Medications don't work well for relieving shortness of breath.

A tracheostomy can be an important part of making you feel comfortable and should be discussed with your physician early on, rather than waiting until it becomes an emergency procedure.

Ideally, your care will be managed by a team of health care professionals. This team can include not only surgeons, medical oncologists, and radiation oncologists but also a social worker, pain specialist, nutritionist, and nurse. All of these specialists bring important skills in helping you to get through this difficult time. Spiritual support is an important part of care for many individuals, and assistance from clergy or religious leaders can prove invaluable. Finally, a diagnosis of incurable cancer should trigger you to get your affairs in order. It is not giving up hope to make sure your will is up to date. Make sure that your family knows where to find bank statements and other assets; it is simply good sense.

SETTING SHORT-TERM GOALS

Though it would be wonderful to make plans for 10 years from now and expect to be here to carry them out, it may not be realistic to do so. Begin with setting short-term goals. Plan to see how effectively the cancer responds to the treatment recommended. Short term goals may be 1 year in length. Discuss with your doctor frankly what to expect. Don't purchase cruise line tickets for 3 years from now in your name that are not refundable. Be optimistic but realistic. Your goal may be to be here in 3 years but first see how your body responds to treatment of the metastasis before making any assumptions. Ask the doctor how long you will undergo treatment before scans will be repeated to see how effective the medications are at shrinking the cancer.

QUALITY OF LIFE VS. QUANTITY OF LIFE

The mission for anyone who has been told their cancer is terminal should be maintaining good quality of life and not just focusing on how many days, weeks, or years you are here. Quantity needs to take a back seat to quality of life. Living a long time in severe pain, unable to take care of your daily needs, and not enjoying still being alive is no way to live. A shorter length of time during which you feel pretty good and are enjoying family is far better than a longer length of time spent miserable. If you are experiencing a lot of pain, speak up. There are a range of medications that control pain. If one stops working, there are other options. Your doctors and nurses may not know that you are suffering if you don't tell them. Sometimes patients are frightened about reporting new symptoms, fearing they will hear that this means the prognosis is worse. There are situations though in which giving a little bit of radiation to the spine, for example, may literally take back pain away completely. This can only happen by telling the doctor your symptoms and how you feel.

WHEN SHOULD I STOP TREATMENT?

The decision about when to stop treatment is not an easy one to make. Having a candid discussion with your doctor about stopping treatment is very valuable. It may require a one-on-one meeting without family present since they may not want to hear the answer to this question. In general, treatment can continue as long as you are responding to treatment, as long as there remain treatment options, and your quality of life is being maintained and not worsened by treatment. There is no sense in doing treatment just for treatment's sake, if it isn't helping. You want your doctor to be very honest and open with you. It will be just as hard for your physician to tell you that he or she recommends stopping treatment as it will be for you to hear those words. Physicians are trained to make patients better and to reduce pain and suffering. Having to tell someone that continuing treatment isn't going to be beneficial is hard, but is important to state if and when such a time comes. Being prepared for such a time is wise. This means asking the doctor how long you can anticipate being able to hold the disease at bay, what drugs can you anticipate being offered and for how long, etc.

Be sure to have your affairs in order and your wishes known. There is a tendency to postpone doing this, perhaps because of denial. Everyone, whether they have cancer or not, should have their affairs in order. Life is unpredictable, and we don't know the future. You are in a situation that is providing you with a window into your future and to see what time line the future holds for you. Take advantage of this unusual knowledge and make sure you have a will, an advanced directive, your finances in order, and your wishes clearly known to your next of kin.

HOSPICE

When we reach the end of life, there are special medical services available to help in preparing for leaving this world, dying with dignity as well as with pain in control, and having you and your family's emotional needs met. Hospice is an organization that helps make this possible and provides support not only for you but for the whole family.

The term hospice derives from medieval times and refers to a place of shelter or rest or "hospitality" to travelers, pilgrims, and the sick and wounded during long journeys. Dame Cicely Saunders at St. Christopher's Hospice in London coined the term "hospice" in 1967 to define specialized care for dying patients and described the hospice approach eloquently: "You matter because of who you are. You matter to the last moment of your life, and we will do all we can, not only to help you die peacefully, but also to live until you die." Today's hospice organizations continue that tradition and provide comprehensive family-centered care that meets not only physical but also social, emotional, and spiritual needs for people in the final phases of incurable disease. Hospice aims to provide comfort and maximize quality of life.

The hospice philosophy accepts death as the final stage of life. Comfort care and symptom relief are the primary focus of hospice care. The goal of hospice is to allow you to have as full and pain-free a life as possible and to manage any other symptoms you might have so that your last days may be spent with dignity, surrounded by your loved ones. Hospice care does not hasten or postpone death. Hospice care treats the person rather than the disease and focuses on quality rather than length of life. The patient and the family are involved in all phases of decision making. Hospice provides equally important supportive care for family members, who may feel overwhelmed by grief, sadness, and the responsibilities of providing care.

Hospice care can be provided in a hospice facility or in your home or in a relative's home. It's your choice. Most people prefer to receive hospice care in their own home and involve family members as caregivers. As your needs change, the hospice providers will adjust pain medications, frequency of visits and care, and if your needs become such that you cannot be cared for comfortably at home, they will arrange admission to an in-patient hospice facility. Unlike typical hospitals, these are usually more home-like and their only goal is to make you comfortable and take care of your needs. Most hospice organizations are family-centered and will involve family members in all aspects of your care. Social services, psychological and spiritual counseling are important parts of hospice care and are provided if desired by the patient and family.

Making initial contact with a hospice program is appropriate when medical treatment is no longer providing any benefit and you are not expected to live for longer than 6 months. To join a hospice program, you must have decided not to pursue any further anti-cancer treatment such as chemotherapy or radiation therapy. A referral from your doctor is needed and is commonly arranged around the time the decision is made that treatment is no longer benefiting you. It is important to remember that hospice care *does not hasten or postpone death*. Hospice is not giving up, but rather making the choice to take back control at the end, when treatment options have been exhausted, to maintain your quality of life for as long as possible, to make the most of each day and spend time where and how you want to spend it, and to be pain-free. If your cancer should go into remission or new treatment options arise, you can always stop hospice and resume treatment. Hospice offers the hope that your quality of life tomorrow will be better than today. This is your chance to make the most of the time you have left, take back control, and to find peace, comfort, and dignity at the end of this storm.

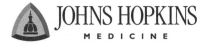

CHAPTER 10

HEAD AND NECK CANCER IN OLDER ADULTS

Gary R. Shapiro, MD

Although head and neck cancers usually occurs in 50 and 60 year olds, as many as 25% are found in those older than 70. As we live longer, the number of people with cancers of the head and neck will increase. In the next 25 years, the number of people who are 65 years of age and older will double, and the largest increases in cancer incidence will occur in those older than 80 years of age.

Older adults with cancer often have other chronic health problems and may be taking multiple medications that can affect their cancer treatment plan. Prejudice, misunderstanding, and limited access to clinical trials often prevent older patients from getting the timely cancer treatment that they need.

Older men and woman may not have adequate screening for head and neck cancer and when a cancer is found, it is too often ignored or undertreated. As a result, older individuals often have more advanced stage cancer and worse outcomes than younger patients.

WHY IS THERE MORE CANCER IN OLDER PEOPLE?

The organs in our body are made up of cells. Cells divide and multiply as the body needs them. Cancer develops when cells in a part of the body grow out of control. The body has a number of ways of repairing damaged control mechanisms, but as we get older, these do not work as well. Although our current healthier lifestyles have allowed us to avoid death from infection, heart attack, and stroke, we may now live long enough for a cancer to develop. People who live longer have increased exposure to cancer-causing agents (carcinogens) in the environment. Aging decreases the body's ability to protect us from these carcinogens and to repair cells that are damaged by these and other processes.

HEAD AND NECK CANCER IS DIFFERENT IN OLDER PEOPLE

Head and neck cancers are more common in men than in women, but among older patients, the percentage of women with head and neck cancer increases. The known environmental risks factors (tobacco, alcohol, sun exposure, occupational inhalants, and HPV and EBV infections) for squamous cell cancers of the head and neck are not as common in older patients as they are in younger patients. Indeed, advanced age itself may be one of the main contributing factors in cancer development. As in younger patients, head and neck cancers usually involve the larynx, oropharynx, or oral cavity. Elderly patients develop more locally advanced (T4) disease but fewer neck lymph node metastases. Elderly patients are also more likely to have additional cancers (second primaries) outside the head and neck region.

DECISION MAKING: 7 PRACTICAL STEPS

1. GET A DIAGNOSIS

No matter how "typical" the signs and symptoms, first impressions are sometimes wrong. That suspicious mass may not be a squamous cell cancer but a lymphoma that, though malignant, requires relatively simple treatment or no treatment at all. It might even be benign. A diagnosis helps you and your family to understand what to expect and how to prepare for the future, even if you cannot get curative treatment. Knowing the diagnosis also helps your doctor treat your symptoms better. Many people find "not knowing" very hard and are relieved when they finally have an explanation for their symptoms. Sometimes a frail patient is obviously dying, and diagnostic studies can be an additional burden. In such cases, it may be quite reasonable to focus on symptom relief (palliation) without knowing the details of the diagnosis.

2. KNOW THE CANCER'S STAGE

The cancer's stage defines your prognosis and treatment options. No one can make informed decisions without it. Just as there may be times when the burdens of diagnostic studies may be too great, it may also be appropriate to do without full staging in very frail, dying patients.

As it is in younger patients, the stage is determined by the size of the tumor, the presence or absence of cancer in lymph nodes, or its spread (metastasis) to other organs. When doctors combine this information with information regarding your cancer's site of origin, they can predict what impact, if any, your head and neck cancer is likely to have on your life expectancy and quality of life.

3. KNOW YOUR LIFE EXPECTANCY

Anti-cancer treatment should be considered if you are likely to live long enough to experience symptoms or premature death from head and neck cancer. If your life expectancy is so short that the cancer will not significantly affect it, there may be no reason to treat your cancer.

However, chronological age (how old you are) should not be the only thing that determines how your cancer should or should not be treated. Despite advanced age, people who are relatively well often have a life expectancy that is longer than their life expectancy with head and neck cancer. The average 70-year-old woman is likely to live another 16 years, and the average 70-year-old man is likely to live another 12 years. A similar 85-year-old can expect to live an additional 5 to 6 years and remain independent for most of that time. Even an unhealthy 75-year-old man or woman probably will live 5 to 6 more years—long enough to suffer symptoms and early death from recurrent head and neck cancer.

4. UNDERSTAND THE GOALS

The Goals of Treatment

It is important to be clear whether the goal of treatment is cure (surgery, radiation therapy, or both combined, with or without adjuvant chemotherapy therapy, for early stage head and neck cancer) or palliation (radiation or chemotherapy for incurable locally advanced or metastatic head and neck cancer). If the goal is palliation, you need to understand if the treatment plan will extend your life, control your symptoms, or both. How likely is it to achieve these goals, and how long will you enjoy their benefits?

When the goal of treatment is palliation, chemotherapy should never be administered without defined endpoints and timelines. It should be clear to everyone what "counts" as success, how it will be determined (for example, a symptom controlled or a smaller mass on a CT scan), and when. You and your family should understand what your options are at each step, and how likely each is to meet your goals. If this is not clear, ask your doctor to explain it in words that you understand.

The Goals of the Patient

In addition to the traditional goals of tumor response, increased survival, and symptom control, older cancer patients often have goals related to quality of life. These may include physical and intellectual independence, spending quality time with family, taking trips, staying out of the hospital, or even economic stability. At times, palliative care or hospice may meet these goals better than active anti-cancer treatment. In addition to the medical team, older patients often turn to family, friends, and clergy to help guide them.

5. DETERMINE IF YOU ARE FIT OR FRAIL

Deciding how to treat cancer in someone who is older requires a thorough understanding of her general health and social situation. Decisions about cancer treatment should never focus on age alone.

Age Is Not a Number

Your actual age (chronological age) has limited influence on how cancer will respond to therapy or its prognosis. Biological and other changes associated with aging are more reliable in estimating an individual's vigor, life expectancy, or the risk of treatment complications. These changes include malnutrition, loss of muscle mass and strength, depression, dementia, falls, social isolation, and the ability to accomplish daily activities such as dressing, bathing, eating, shopping, housekeeping, and managing one's finances or medication.

Chronic Illnesses

Older cancer patients are likely to have chronic illnesses (comorbidity) that affect their life expectancy; the more illnesses you have, the greater the effect. This effect has very little impact on the behavior of the cancer itself, but studies do show that comorbidity has a major impact on treatment outcome and its side effects.

6. BALANCE BENEFITS AND HARMS

Fit older head and neck cancer patients respond to treatment similarly to their younger counterparts. However, a word of caution is in order. Until recently, few studies included older individuals, and it may not be appropriate to apply these findings to the diverse group of older cancer patients.

The side effects of cancer treatment are never less in the elderly. In addition to the standard side effects, there are significant age-related toxicities to consider. Though most of these are more a function of frailty than chronological age, even the fittest senior cannot avoid the physical effects of aging. In addition to the changes in fat and muscle that you see in the mirror, there are age-related changes in your kidney, liver, and digestive (gastrointestinal) function. These changes affect how your body absorbs and metabolizes anti-cancer drugs and other medicines. The average senior takes many different medicines (to control, for example, high blood pressure, high cholesterol, osteoporosis, diabetes, arthritis, etc.). This "polypharmacy" can cause undesirable side effects as the many drugs interact with each other and the anti-cancer medications.

7. GET INVOLVED

Health care providers and family members often underestimate the physical and mental abilities of older people and their willingness to face chronic and life-threatening conditions. Studies clearly show that older patients want detailed and easily understood information about potential treatments and alternatives. Patients and families may consider cancer untreatable in the aged and not understand the possibilities offered by treatment.

Although patients with dementia pose a unique challenge, they are frequently capable of participating in goal setting and simple discussions about treatment side effects and logistics. Caring family members and friends are often able to share the patient's life story so that health care workers can work with them to make decisions consistent with the patient's values and desires. This of course is no substitute for a well thought out and properly executed living will or healthcare proxy.

While it is hard to face the possibility of life-threatening events at any age, it is always better to be prepared and to put your affairs in order. In addition to estate planning and wills, it is critical that you outline your wishes regarding medical care at the end of life, and make legal provisions for someone to make those decisions if you are unable to make them for yourself.

TREATING HEAD AND NECK CANCER

YOU NEED A TEAM

Cancer care changes rapidly, and it is hard for the generalist to keep up to date so referral to a specialist is essential. The needs of an older cancer patient often extend beyond the doctor's office and the traditional services provided by visiting nurses. These needs may include transportation, nutrition, and emotional, financial, physical, or spiritual support. When an older woman or man with head and neck cancer is the primary care giver for a frail or ill spouse, grandchildren, or other family members, special attention is necessary to provide for their needs as well. Older cancer patients cared for in geriatric oncology programs benefit from multidisciplinary teams of oncologists, geriatricians, psychiatrists, pharmacists, physiatrists, social workers, nurses, clergy, and dieticians all working together as a team to identify and manage the stressors that can limit effective cancer treatment.

SURGERY

Though head and neck cancer surgery is often complex, it is the standard of care for most early-stage cancers of the head and neck, regardless of age (see Chapter 3). Like other treatment options, surgery in some older individuals may involve risks related to decreases in body organ function, especially the heart and lungs. It is essential that the surgeon and anesthesiologist work closely with your primary care physician (or a consultant) to fully assess and treat these problems before, during, and after the operation.

Surgery is as effective in elderly patients as in younger patients, but it does have a somewhat higher rate of complications in older individuals who have other medical problems (comorbidities). Since radiation therapy and chemotherapy often have even higher risks, they are usually no substitute for surgery. If an older person is too frail to undergo curative surgery, he is usually too frail to get curative radiation or chemotherapy. There are a few exceptions to this general rule, and it is essential that you weigh all of the risks and benefits with your multidisciplinary care team.

Free flap reconstructive surgery is somewhat controversial in the elderly, but a number of recent studies show that this microvascular procedure is a safe and reliable option in the great majority of older patients (see Chapter 3). The risk of complications is due more to an individual patient's coexisting illnesses, especially cardiovascular disease, than to her age or the duration of the operation. However, even in the absence of significant comorbidity, microvascular reconstruction in those over 80 years old is often associated with increased complications and monetary cost.

RADIATION THERAPY

Radiation therapy is rarely the treatment of choice for early-stage cancer of the head and neck. Sometimes doctors use it in combination with chemotherapy to treat stage 1 or 2 cancer of the oral cavity, but surgery is usually more effective and actually has fewer side effects. It is an essential post-operative adjunct for most stage 3 or 4 head and neck cancers, and doctors often recommended it for earlier stage tumors with aggressive pathology (see Chapter 3). They may also add sensitizing chemotherapy in these situations.

In two-thirds of people with stage 3 larynx cancer the non-operative approach preserves the larynx (and thus the natural voice), and the side effects of chemoradiation therapy may be worth it. However, some older larynx cancer patients with limited mobility or difficulties with transportation may prefer surgery to the frequent visits to the hospital required for radiation and chemotherapy. The effect of radiation on swallowing function is more severe in the elderly, particularly when chemoradiation is used and some older larynx cancer patients with pre-existing swallowing trouble do better with a surgical approach. Similar quality of life decisions usually weigh in favor of non-operative chemoradiation therapy when it comes to treating cancer of the base of the tongue.

Radiation therapy-induced mouth sores (mucositis) and dry mouth (xerostomia) can be more problematic in older patients who are already at risk for dehydration and malnutrition, but dehydration, weight loss, and electrolyte disturbances can be avoided with careful monitoring and early treatment. Regular, meticulous inspection of the mouth with prompt treatment to control pain and infection is essential. The early use of topical moisturizing agents can minimize skin toxicity.

Radiation therapy usually provides excellent symptom relief (palliation) in metastatic and other incurable situations. It is also often quite effective in cancers that have recurred after initial surgery. It is particularly effective in treating pain caused by head and neck cancer metastases to the bone. A short course of radiation therapy often allows patients with advanced cancer to lower (or even eliminate) their dose of narcotic pain relievers. Although these medicines do an excellent job of controlling pain, they often cause confusion, falls, and constipation in older patients. Thus, even hospice patients suffering from localized metastatic bone pain should consider the option of palliative radiation therapy.

The fatigue that usually accompanies radiation therapy can be quite profound in the elderly, even in those who are fit. Often the logistical details (like daily travel to the hospital for a 6-week course of treatment) are the hardest for older people. It is important that you discuss these potential problems with your family and social worker, prior to starting radiation therapy.

CHEMOTHERAPY

Non-frail older cancer patients respond to chemotherapy similarly to their younger counterparts. Reducing the dose of chemotherapy (or radiation therapy) based purely on chronological age may seriously affect the effectiveness of treatment. Managing chemotherapy-associated toxicity with appropriate supportive care is crucial in the elderly population to give them the best chance of cure and survival or to provide the best palliation.

The addition of cisplatin to adjuvant radiotherapy after surgery is beneficial when extracapsular spread or positive margins are present (see Chapter 3). However, the magnitude of this benefit is greatest in those aged 60 or less, who may be better able to tolerate the side effects of chemotherapy. This benefit is not without its down side. Older patients have a higher rate of mouth sores (mucositis), diarrhea, thrombocytopenia (low platelet blood count that can cause bleeding), and kidney (nephrotoxicity) side effects. Severe side effects are more common in cisplatin-based chemotherapy programs than those that use other drugs. There is little information available about the risks and benefits of Erbitux (cetuximab) in older patients with head and neck cancer.

Though the side effects of cancer treatment are never less burdensome in the elderly, they can be managed by oncologists, especially geriatric oncologists, who work in teams with others who specialize in the care of the elderly. With appropriate care, healthy older patients do just as well with chemotherapy as younger patients. Advances in supportive care (anti-nausea medicines and blood cell growth factors) have significantly decreased the side effects of chemotherapy and improved safety and the quality of life of individuals with head and neck cancer. Nonetheless, there is risk, especially if the patient is frail. The presence of severe comorbidities, age-related frailty, or underlying severe psychosocial problems may be obstacles for highly intensive treatment plans. Such patients may benefit from less complicated or potentially less toxic treatment plans.

COMMON TREATMENT COMPLICATIONS IN THE ELDERLY

Anemia (low red blood cell count) is common in the elderly, especially the frail elderly. Anemia decreases the effectiveness of chemotherapy and often causes fatigue, falls, cognitive decline (for example, dementia, disorientation, or confusion), and heart problems. Therefore, it is essential that anemia be recognized and corrected with red blood cell transfusions or the appropriate use of erythropoiesis-stimulating agents like epoetin (Procrit, Epogen) or darbepoetin (Aranesp).

Myelosuppression (low white blood cell count) is also common in older patients getting chemotherapy or radiation therapy. Older patients with myelosuppression develop life-threatening infections more often than younger patients, and they may need to be treated in the hospital for many days. The liberal use of granulopoietic growth factors (G-CSF, Neupogen, Neulasta) decreases the risk of infection and makes it possible for older women to receive full doses of potentially curable adjuvant chemotherapy.

Mucositis (mouth sores) and **diarrhea** can cause severe **dehydration** in older patients who often are already dehydrated due to inadequate fluid intake and diuretics ("water pills" for high blood pressure or heart failure). Careful monitoring and the liberal use of anti-diarrheal agents (Imodium) and oral and intravenous fluids are essential components of the management of older cancer patients, especially those receiving head and neck radiation or 5-fluorouracil (5-FU) or both.

Xerostomia (dry mouth) may also contribute to dehydration and malnutrition in older head and neck cancer patients. Older patients occasionally have a harder time adapting to dry mouth and other functional disabilities that follow operative and non-operative treatments, in particular the swallowing problems (**dysphagia**) that can result from radiation therapy. Many older patients go to nursing homes for several weeks after treatment and often do not get adequate rehabilitation and swallowing therapy.

Kidney function declines as we age. Some of the medicines that older patients take to treat both their cancer (cisplatin, carboplatin, NSAIDs) and non-cancer-related problems might make kidney function worse. The dehydration that often accompanies cancer and its treatment can put additional stress on the kidneys. Fortunately, it is often possible to minimize these effects by carefully selecting and dosing appropriate drugs, managing "polypharmacy," and preventing dehydration.

Neurotoxicity and **cognitive effects ("chemo-brain")** can be profoundly debilitating in patients who are already cognitively impaired (demented, disoriented, confused, etc.). Elderly patients with a history of falling, hearing loss, or peripheral neuropathy (nerve damage from, for example, diabetes) have decreased energy and are highly vulnerable to neurotoxic chemotherapy like the taxanes or platinum compounds. Many of the medicines used to control nausea (anti-emetics) or decrease the side effects of certain chemotherapeutic agents are also potential neurotoxins. These include dexamethasone (psychosis and agitation), ranitidine (agitation), diphenhydramine, and some of the anti-emetics (sedation).

Fatigue is a near universal complaint of older cancer patients. It is particularly a problem for those who are socially isolated or depend upon others to help them with activities of daily living. Fatigue is not necessarily related to **depression**, but it can be. Depression is quite common in the elderly. In contrast to younger patients who often respond to a cancer diagnosis with anxiety, depression is the more common disorder in older cancer patients. With proper support and medical attention, many of these patients can safely receive anti-cancer treatment.

Heart problems increase with age, and it is no surprise that older cancers patients have an increased risk of cardiac complications from intensive surgery, radiation, and chemotherapy. Patients treated with cisplatin chemotherapy require large amounts of intravenous fluid hydration. This can cause congestive heart failure in patients with heart problems; they need careful monitoring. **Atherosclero-**

sis (blood vessel damage form hardening of the arteries) may increase the chances of local radiation therapy toxicity or make microvascular free flap reconstructive surgery more difficult.

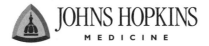

CHAPTER 11

TRUSTED RESOURCES—FINDING ADDITIONAL INFORMATION ABOUT HEAD AND NECK CANCER AND ITS TREATMENT

Erin J. Blume, BS, RHIA
Christine G. Gourin, MD, FACS

A cancer diagnosis brings many questions and a need for clear, understandable answers. A multitude of organizations and web sites exists for cancer patients; the resources listed below provide more detailed information and support services to help you manage head and neck cancer. An informed patient is an empowered patient.

ORGANIZATIONS

The following are national organizations that provide information and support for people with head and neck cancer.

AMERICAN CANCER SOCIETY

Toll-free: 800–ACS–2345 (800–227–3345)

Web site: www.cancer.org

The American Cancer Society is the nationwide community-based voluntary health organization dedicated to eliminating cancer as a major health problem by preventing cancer, saving lives, and diminishing suffering from cancer through research, education, advocacy, and service. The American Cancer Society web site contains information about many of the challenges of cancer and survivorship. You can search for information by cancer type or by topic. ACS provides a list of support groups in your area or you can join online groups and message boards.

AMERICAN HEAD AND NECK SOCIETY

Web site: www.ahns.info

The American Head and Neck Society (AHNS) is the single largest organization in North America for the advancement of research and education in head and neck oncology. The AHNS supports Fellowships in Advanced Training in Head & Neck Oncologic Surgery, which must meet strict criteria for training head and neck cancer surgeons and offers links to clinical trial resources and clinical practice guidelines on their website.

CANCER*CARE*, INC.

Toll-free: 800–813–HOPE (800–813–4673)

Web site: www.cancercare.org

Cancer*Care* is a national nonprofit organization that provides free, professional support services to anyone affected by cancer—people with cancer, caregivers, children, loved ones, and the bereaved. Cancer*Care* programs—including counseling, education, financial assistance and practical help—are provided by trained oncology social workers and are completely free of charge. A comprehensive list of online support groups is available at their website.

CANCER.NET

Web site: www.cancer.net

Cancer.Net, formerly People Living With Cancer (PLWC), brings the expertise and resources of the American Society of Clinical Oncology (ASCO), the voice of the world's cancer physicians, to people living with cancer and those who care for and care about them. All the information and content on Cancer.Net was developed and approved by the cancer doctors who are members of ASCO, making Cancer. Net the most up-to-date and trusted resource for cancer information on the Internet. Cancer.Net provides timely, oncologist-approved information to help patients and families make informed health care decisions.

INTERNATIONAL ASSOCIATION OF LARYNGECTOMEES (IAL)

Web site: www.theial.com

The International Association of Laryngectomees (IAL) is a nonprofit voluntary organization composed of approximately 250 member clubs and recognized regional organizations. These clubs are generally known as "Lost Chord" or "New Voice" clubs comprised of anywhere from 10 to more than 300 Laryngectomees. The purpose of the IAL is to assist these local clubs in their efforts toward the total rehabilitation of the Laryngectomee.

NATIONAL CANCER INSTITUTE (NCI)

Toll-free: 800–4–CANCER (800–422–6237)

TTY (tele typewriter): 800–332–8615

Web site: www.cancer.gov

Cancer.gov, the National Cancer Institute web site, provides accurate, up-to-date information on many types of cancer and the challenges cancer can bring. You can also use the site to search for information by cancer type or topic, and you can access information about treatment-related issues. Information about financial and insurance matters is also included. You can learn how clinical trials work and search for a clinical trial in your area. This site has a detailed dictionary of cancer terms.

NATIONAL COMPREHENSIVE CANCER NETWORK

Web site: www.nccn.com

The National Comprehensive Cancer Network (NCCN) is a non-profit alliance of 21 major cancer centers. The NCCN provides clinical practice guidelines for cancer treatment by site and valuable resources for patients about managing symptoms, your legal rights at work, prescription and travel assistance, paying for treatment, and wellness for surviors.

SUPPORT FOR PATIENTS WITH ORAL AND HEAD AND NECK CANCER (SPOHNC)

Web site: www.spohnc.org

SPOHNC is a patient-directed, self-help organization dedicated to meeting the needs of oral and head and neck cancer patients. SPOHNC, founded in 1991 by an oral cancer survivor, addresses the broad emotional, physical, and humanistic needs of this population. SPHONC provides a list of support groups in your area.

THE HEAD AND NECK CANCER ALLIANCE

Toll–free: 843–792–6624

Web site: www.headandneck.org

The mission of this organization is to provide support to head and neck cancer patients throughout the year, educate children and adults in the disease process, treatment, and prevention of head and neck cancer, and support ongoing research in head and neck oncology. This Foundation was originally created by the generosity of actor Yul Brynner following successful treatment of a precancerous larynx growth in 1983.

WEBWHISPERS

Web site: www.webwhispers.org

WebWhispers was started in 1996 for those who had questions about larynx cancer treatments, surgery, recovery, and what life is like after laryngectomy surgery. WebWhispers is now the largest support group for individual laryngec-tomee survivors of larynx and other throat cancers. Web-Whispers offers advice from those who have been there and education at the time it is needed. WebWhispers members support patients in their rehabilitation.

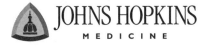

INFORMATION ABOUT
JOHNS HOPKINS

Johns Hopkins Head and Neck Cancer Center
http://headneckcancer.hopkinskimmelcancercenter.org

The Johns Hopkins Head and Neck Cancer Center provides comprehensive care in treatment and post-treatment services for patients with head and neck cancer as well as access to the latest and most promising therapies. Our multidisciplinary approach to head and neck cancer care ensures that patients have access to specialists in every aspect of their disease, and that treatment planning takes into account all facets of their care and considers the entire range of treatment options. The team also includes professionals who can help patients and their families to cope with the emotional and practical aspects of disease and related issues such as smoking cessation.

Sidney Kimmel Comprehensive Cancer Center at Johns Hopkins

http://www.hopkinskimmelcancercenter.org

Since its inception in 1973, the Sidney Kimmel Comprehensive Cancer Center at Johns Hopkins has been dedicated to better understanding human cancers and finding more effective treatments. One of only forty cancer centers in the country designated by the National Cancer Institute (http://www.cancer.gov) as a Comprehensive Cancer Center, the Johns Hopkins Kimmel Cancer Center has active programs in clinical research, laboratory research, education, community outreach, and prevention and control, and is the only Comprehensive Cancer Center in the state of Maryland.

About Johns Hopkins Medicine

http://www.hopkinsmedicine.org

Johns Hopkins Medicine unites physicians and scientists of the Johns Hopkins University School of Medicine with the organizations, health professionals, and facilities of the Johns Hopkins Health System. Its mission is to improve the health of the community and the world by setting the standard of excellence in medical education, research, and clinical care. Diverse and inclusive, Johns Hopkins Medicine has provided international leadership in the education of physicians and medical scientists in biomedical research and in the application of medical knowledge to sustain health since The Johns Hopkins Hospital opened in 1889.

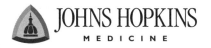

FURTHER READING

100 Questions & Answers About Esophageal Cancer, Second Edition, Pamela K. Ginex, EdD, RN, OCN, Maureen Jingeleski, RN, BSN, Bart L. Frazzitta, and Manjit S. Bains, MD, Jones & Bartlett Learning, 2010.

100 Questions & Answers About Gastric Cancer, Manish A. Shah, MD, Natasha A. Pinheiro, RN, BSN, Brinda Shawh, RPh, Jones & Bartlett Learning, 2008.

100 Questions & Answers About Thyroid Disorders, Warner M. Burch, MD, Jones & Bartlett Learning, 2009.

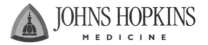

GLOSSARY

Adenocarcinoma: A malignant tumor that most commonly arises in salivary gland tissue or the esophagus, though it can also arise in the sinuses.

Advanced-stage cancer: *See* staging.

Anaplastic: Of or characterized by cells that have become less differentiated.

Benign: Not malignant; self-limiting.

Biopsy: The removal for diagnostic study of a piece of tissue from a living body.

Breslow system: Used as a prognostic factor in melanoma of the skin. It is a description of how deeply tumor cells have invaded.

CAT scan: An examination performed using a CAT scanner; also called CT scan.

Cervical esophagus: The upper-third of the esophagus, considered part of the head and neck.

Chemoradiation: Chemotherapy plus radiation given together.

Chemotherapy: Refers to drugs that are cytotoxic. That is, they cause cell death. There are many different types of chemotherapy drugs, all with different mechanisms of action that result in tumor cell death.

Clinical trials: Research studies in which people agree to try new therapies under careful supervision in order to help doctors identify the best treatments with the fewest side effects.

Duct: A tube, canal, or vessel conveying a body fluid, especially a glandular secretion or excretion.

Early-stage cancer: Cancer which has not spread to lymph nodes and is small; *see also* staging.

Endoscope: A slender, tubular optical instrument used as a viewing system for examining an inner part of the body and can be used for biopsy or surgery.

Erbitux: A monoclonal antibody that binds to the epidermal growth factor receptor (EGFR).

Epstein Barr virus (EBV): A type of herpes virus that causes infectious mononucleosis.

Esophagus: Starts just below the larynx and carries food through the chest to the stomach.

Extracapsular spread: Infiltration of cancer cells beyond the capsule of a metastatic lymph node.

Hospice: A health-care facility for the terminally ill that emphasizes pain control and emotional support for the patient and family, typically refraining from taking extraordinary measures to prolong life.

Human papillomavirus (HPV): Any of various strains of papovirus that cause warts, especially of the hands, feet, and genitals, with some strains believed to be a causative factor in cancer of the cervix, tonsil, and tongue base.

Hypopharynx: The back wall of the digestive tract below the tongue and behind the larynx, including the upper part of the esophagus, also called the cervical esophagus.

Larynx: "Voice box"; the true vocal cords, false vocal cords above the true vocal cords, epiglottis or valve above the vocal cords that protects you from food being swallowed into your lungs, and the trachea or windpipe immediately below the vocal cords, with surrounding cartilage ("Adam's apple").

Lymph nodes: Gland-like masses of tissue in the lymphatic vessels containing cells that become lymphocytes. There are hundreds of lymph nodes in both sides of the neck; these contain lymphatic tissue, which filter foreign substances and make white blood cells.

Lymphedema: Swelling in your face and jaw, common after neck surgery.

Lymphoma: A cancer that arises from lymphoid tissue. It can arise anywhere within the head and neck.

Malignant: Characterized by uncontrolled growth; cancerous, invasive, or metastatic.

Merkel cell cancer: A very rare skin cancer that manifests aggressive behavior with a high incidence of spread to other sites in the body.

MRI: Magnetic resonance imaging; a noninvasive diagnostic procedure employing an MR scanner to obtain detailed sectional images of the internal structure of the body.

Mucoepidermoid carcinoma: This tumor is not encapsulated and is characterized by squamous cells, mucus-secreting cells, and intermediate cells. Generally, there is a good prognosis for low-grade tumors, and a poor prognosis for high-grade tumors.

Mucositis: Inflammation of the mucosal tissues lining the oral cavity and upper digestive tract. A common side effect of radiation, particularly when radiation is combined with chemotherapy.

Multimodality therapy: More than one kind of treatment administered together.

Nasal cavity: Nose.

Nasopharynx: The area behind the nasal passages, at the base of the skull.

Neck: Connects the head and the trunk. In addition to lymph nodes, the neck contains blood vessels and nerves which may give rise to a variety of unusual tumor types.

Neck dissection: A term for lymph node removal.

Node-negative: No evidence of enlarged lymph nodes on examination.

Node-positive: When patients with head and neck cancer have enlarged lymph nodes that can be palpated on examination.

Non-operative therapy: Refers to radiation or chemoradiation.

Oncology: The branch of medical science dealing with tumors, including the origin, development, diagnosis, and treatment of malignant neoplasms; the study of cancer.

Oral cavity: Gums, lips, tongue, area under the tongue or floor of mouth, palate, or roof of the mouth.

Oropharynx: Tonsils, base of the tongue, back wall of the throat at the level of the tongue, the soft palate, and uvula.

Otolaryngology: The branch of medicine that deals with the anatomy, function, and diseases of the ear, nose, and throat.

Palpate: To examine by touch, especially for the purpose of diagnosing disease or illness.

Paragangliomas: These are rare tumors that arise from nerves in the neck or at the base of the skull or from the carotid artery. Surgery is the mainstay of therapy, as these tumors are not sensitive to radiation or chemotherapy.

Parotid glands: Salivary glands that fill out our cheeks.

Passy-Muir valve: This one-way valve attaches to the outside opening of the tracheostomy tube and allows air to pass into the tracheostomy but not out through it. The patient breathes out through the mouth and nose instead of the tracheostomy.

Percutaneous gastrostomy tube (PEG): An endoscopic procedure for placing a tube into the stomach. An alternative to surgical gastrostomy, PEG involves placing a tube into the stomach through the abdominal wall.

Perineural invasion: Refers to cancer that has spread along nerves.

PET scan: Positron emission tomography (PET) is a nuclear medicine imaging technique that produces a three-dimensional image or picture of functional processes in the body.

Primary closure: When the surrounding tissue can be closed over a surgical defect.

Prognosis: A forecasting of the probable course and outcome of a disease, with respect to the chances of cure.

Radiation therapy: The medical use of ionizing radiation as part of cancer treatment to control malignant cells (not to be confused with radiology, the use of radiation in medical imaging and diagnosis).

Radiolabelled isotope (tracer): A technique for tracking the passage of a sample of substance through a system. The substance is "labeled" by including radionuclides in its chemical composition.

Resectable: Capable of being resected; resectable cancer.

Salivary glands: The parotid glands, submandibular glands, and minor salivary glands lining the mouth and throat that make saliva.

Sarcomas: Rare tumors that can arise anywhere within the head and neck.

Sentinel node biopsy: A minimally invasive procedure in which a lymph node near the site of a cancerous tumor is first identified as a sentinel node and then removed for microscopic analysis.

Secondary closure: When there is not enough tissue to close a surgical defect, small areas can be left open to close spontaneously through new tissue from the edges growing in.

Sinuses: Air-filled spaces behind your cheeks, nose, and forehead.

Sinus cancer: Sinus cancers typically arise from the lining of the sinus, a tissue known as mucosa. Early symptoms of sinus cancer are nosebleeds (either blood-streaked nasal mucus, or recurrent "gushers"), tooth pain and a persistently obstructed (stuffy) nose.

Skin cancer: Can refer to all skin involving the head and neck area, including the face, scalp, ears, and neck.

Speech pathology: The field of study of speech and swallowing disorders such as stuttering and dysphasia. Speech pathologists treat speech and swallowing disorders.

Squamous cell carcinoma: A carcinoma that arises from squamous epithelium and is the most common form of skin and head and neck cancer.

Staging: Refers to the extent of the tumor and its spread. Cancer staging systems describe how far cancer has spread anatomically and attempt to put patients with similar prognosis and treatment in the same staging group. Prognosis and treatment depend quite a bit on the stage.

Stoma: An opening created after laryngectomy by attaching the remaining windpipe, or trachea, to the skin.

Submandibular glands: Paired salivary glands located just below our jaw.

Thyroid gland: A butterfly-shaped gland in the lower neck, in front of the larynx, which makes thyroid hormone, important in metabolism.

The TNM stage (tumor, nodes, metastases): System used to stage tumors based on the size of the primary tumor, the degree of lymph node involvement, and the presence or absence of distant metastases.

Trachea: Starts below the larynx; a passage for air to the lungs. Also referred to as the "windpipe".

Tracheostomy: The construction of an artificial opening through the neck into the trachea, usually for the relief of difficulty in breathing.

Tumor grade: A descriptive term referring to the appearance of tumor cells. Numbers 1, 2, or 3 to refer to grade or simply say "low grade" (grades 1 and 2) or "high grade"

(grade 3). Some pathologists use the term "intermediate grade" to refer to grade 2 tumors.

Ultrasound: The application of ultrasonic waves to therapy or diagnostics, as in deep-heat treatment of a joint or imaging of internal structures.

Unresectable cancer: Refers to cancer that invades structures such as the prevertebral muscles of the spine, the carotid artery, the base of the skull, the chest, or the brain.

Xerostomia: Dry mouth, which is a common side effect after radiation and sometimes after surgery.

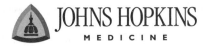

JOHNS HOPKINS
M E D I C I N E

Note: Italicized page locators indicate a figure; tables are noted with a *t*.

Nutrition, 203. *See also* Diet;
Eating; Feeding tube;
Swallowing difficulties
good, 90, 100–101, 141
for older adults, 172
palliative care and, 158
radiation treatment and, 71–73
recovery and, 213–214
Nutritionists, 141
feeding tube management and, 61
incurable cancer and, 159

O

Obturator, tracheostomy tube, 94
"Occult," or microscopic cancer,
in lymph nodes, 11
Occupational inhalants, 166
Older adults
decision making for: 7 practical
steps, 167–172
balancing benefits and harms,
171
determining if you are fit or
frail, 170
get involved, 171
getting a diagnosis, 167
know cancer's stage, 167–168
know your life expectancy, 168
understanding goals of treatment, 169–170
head and neck cancer different
in, 166–167
head and neck cancer in, 165–180
medical team for, 172
treatment complications in,
177–180
anemia, 177
dehydration, 178
fatigue, 179
heart problems, 179–180
kidney function, 178
mucositis, 178
myelosuppression, 177–178

neurotoxicity and cognitive
effects, 179
xerostomia, 178
Older children, talking about
your cancer with, 123–124
Oncology nurses, 6
Oncology team, selecting, 5–8
Online resources, 128
Online support groups, 112, 256
Oral cancer treatment, descrip-
tion of, 203
Oral cavity cancer, 8, 167
recurrences and, 151
surgery for, 42
Oral communication, post-surgery,
218
Oral health and hygiene, 135
importance of, 107
in older cancer patients, 175
Oral prostheses, 58
Oral rinses, 70
Oropharyngeal tumors, advanced,
treatment options for, 45
Oropharynx cancer
early-stage, surgery and, 43
in older patients, 167
Osteoporosis medications, older
patients and, 171
Osteoradionecrosis, 73, 74, 75,
92, 107
Otolaryngologist, 29
Outer cannula, tracheostomy
tube, 94
Ovarian cancer, genetic link in, 2

P

PACU. *See* Post-anesthesia unit
Pain management
goal of, 157
hospice and, 162
incurable cancer and, 155, 156, 157
medications for, 61
quality of life and, 160